CBD Hemp Oil

50 Proven Ways Natural CBD Oil Can Rejuvenate Your Body And Restore Your Health

By Mary Jones

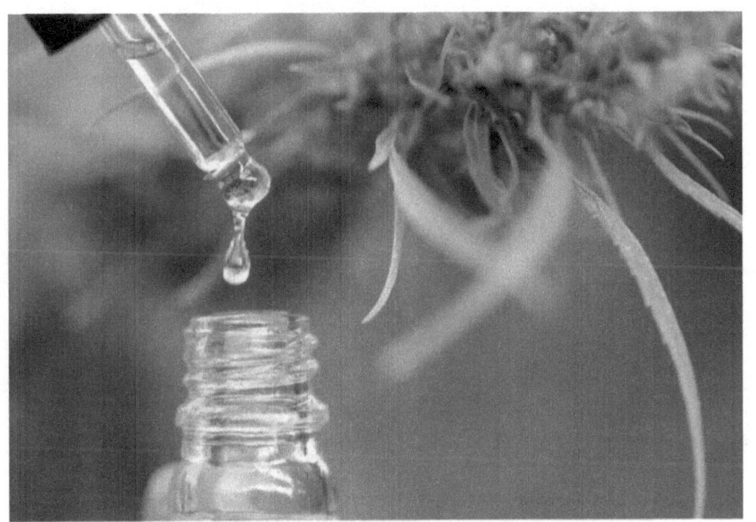

*"Using CBD Oil for your self-care practice can be
a powerful way to create change and care for yourself."*

TABLE OF CONTENTS

INTRODUCTION

In a world where more and more people are turning to complementary medicines, rising to 33.2% of the population in the US alone in 2012, CBD – or cannabidiol – is getting an increasing amount of attention, and for very good reason too! According to **Gallup data** of 2019 (at _gallup.com_), *14% of Americans say they use CBD Products*. As this book will show you, the benefits that you can gain from using this oil are seemingly endless!

Now, the name of the oil can put some people off because they immediately think of the illegal substance, cannabis, but this oil is simply extracted from the resin glands on the marijuana bud, or hemp, ensuring that *none* of the inherent illegal substances are included. The part that's associated with getting people 'high' is tetrahydrocannabinol, or THC, which is kept completely separate.

It is suggested that this increase in usage might have something to do with all the **ailments that can be helped or even cured using CBD**, as this book will extensively show you.

These ailments include:

- Pain
- Mental Illness
- Sickness
- Neurological Disorders
- Cardiovascular Health

To name just a few. In fact, as you will go on to read, there aren't many ailments that can't be helped with CBD; although, of course, any information given in this book is not to be taken as medical advice. You will also need to consult your doctor to get the best, individual advice for you.

Not only will this book tell you all you need to know about hemp oil, you'll also learn about the science behind it, how they differ, the best application methods, and what to look for when buying. You won't be able to find a more extensive guide than this one!

So, read on to discover how this incredible oil can help you, and become one of the millions of people using it to help with their everyday lives and any illnesses. Whether you suffer from something big and life-altering or something small, there will be information in the following chapters for you.

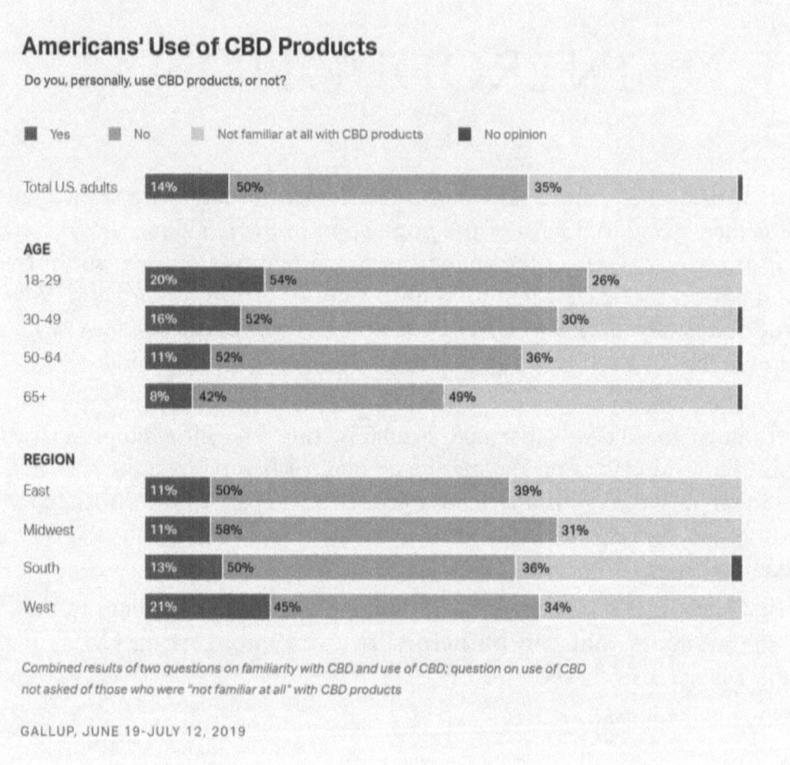

ALL YOU NEED TO KNOW ABOUT HEMP

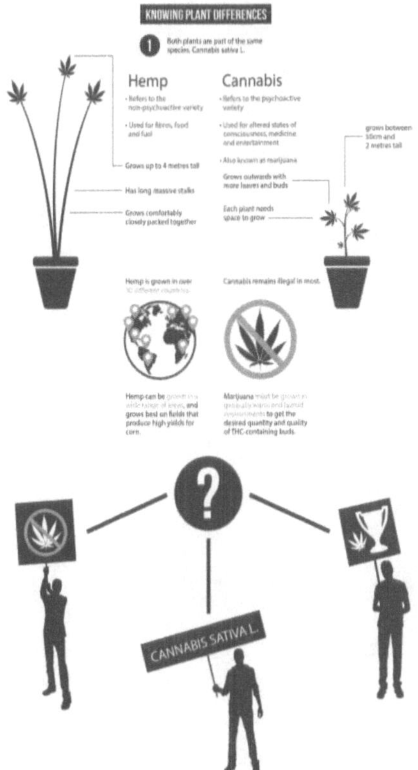

The hemp plant has been used since the agricultural revolution for all kinds of things. The fiber from the plant is used to create things, such as rope, textiles, and paper, used in everyday life. In fact, one of the oldest relics of human history is a scrap of hemp fabric from 8,000 BC.

This chapter will look at the parts of the plant used for medication so you can get to know it a little bit better.

Hemp Seed

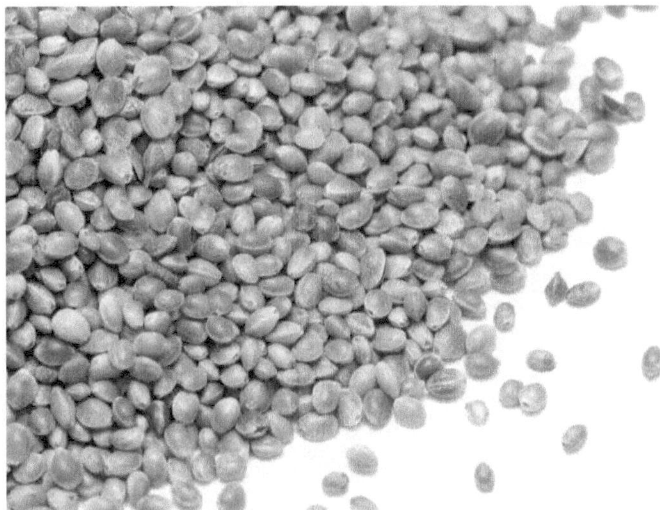

The hemp seed, which the plant grows from, is edible and used for bread, grains, cakes, and many other foods. It's also used to create fuel, lubricants, and ink. While they might not be used directly for medicinal purposes, eating them is said to have **a lot of positive side effects, including these**:

- The Gamma-Linolenic acid (GLA) helps build muscles and control inflammation.

- Studies have shown they're great for arthritis and joint pain.

- The seeds are an appetite suppressant, which assists weight loss.

- They also contain probiotics to aid digestion, keeping your gastrointestinal system regular.

- Eating them regularly will help your hair, skin, and nails look better.

- GLA plus the seed's omega-3 fats will help your immune system.

- Hemp seeds contain key ingredients to promote heart health.

28 grams, or 1 ounce, of hemp seeds consists of:

- 161 calories

- 12.3 g fat

- 3.3 g carbohydrates

- 2.8 mg manganese (140% DV)

- 2 g fiber

- 9.2 g protein

- 15.4 mg vitamin E (77% DV)
- 3.9 mg iron (22% DV)
- 0.1 mg copper (7% DV)
- 5 mg zinc (34% DV)
- 300 mg magnesium (75% DV)
- 405 mg phosphorus (41% DV)

Hemp Oil

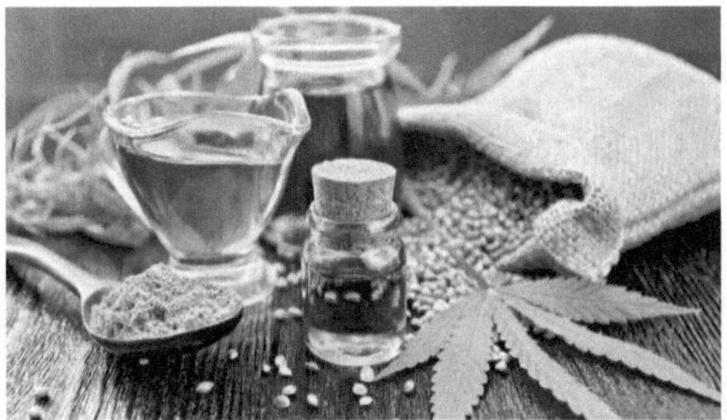

Hemp oil is obtained by pressing hemp seeds. This comes out in a green color; the darker it is, the grassier the flavor. As well as being used for medicinal purposes, it's also great for making soaps, shampoos, and other healthy living products. It can also be used in cooking and to make biodegradable plastic, which makes it safer for the environment.

Here are **the most significant health benefits of hemp oil**:

- Helps to maintain hormone balance.

- It regenerates and energizes the skin's protective layer.

- It helps vegans and vegetarians maintain a healthy ratio of omega-6 and omega-3 fatty acids.

- The Oil helps to lower cholesterol.

- Due to its low carbohydrate and sugar content, hemp oil can be great for diabetics.

- Your immune system will be boosted, which helps with many illnesses.

- It'll also stop things such as varicose veins.

So, while hemp is in the same family as marijuana, it isn't anything like the banned substance. As shown by this guide:

	Cannabis?	Chemical Makeup	Mind-altering?	Agriculture	Uses
Hemp	Yes	THC (less than 0.3%)	No	Needs minimal care. Can adapt to most climates.	Cars, body care, fabric, plastic, construction, food.
Marijuana	Yes	THC (between 5% and 35%)	Yes	Requires carefully controlled climate.	Medicinal, recreational uses

CBD

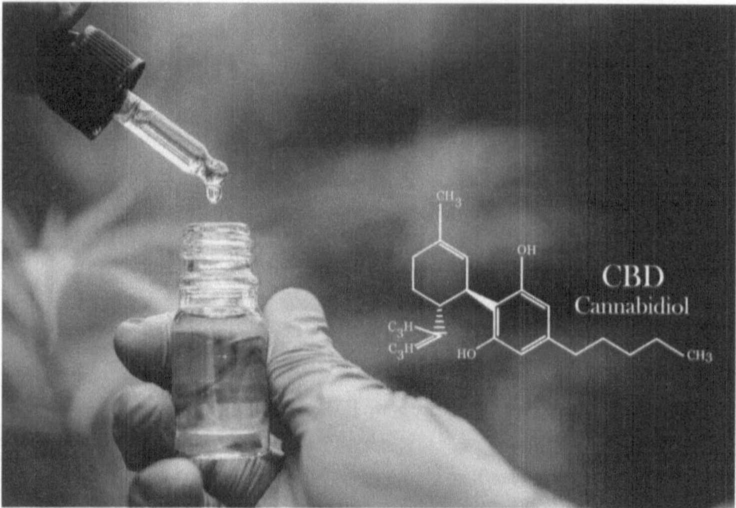

Cannabidiol is a cannabis compound that has significant medical benefits *without* the THC, which causes the psychoactive effects. The lack of those illegal elements is what makes it much better for you. You can receive **all the benefits** listed in this book, without any of the negative.

It can be made from hemp resin and replaces parts of our diets that are often missing, such as vitamins, minerals, proteins, flavonoids, terpenes, and omega fatty acids. For more information on how CBD is sourced, check out **Healthy Hemp Oil** (at *healthyhempoil.com/cannabidiol*).

So, what is in this oil?

CBD oil is cannabis oil that **has a significant content of cannabidiol**. It is made from the flowers, stalks, and leaves of hemp, while hemp oil is made from hemp seeds.

The hemp extract takes up 40% of the CBD oil, and **the rest of it is made up of:**

- Amino acids
- Beta-carotene
- Carbohydrates
- Alkanes
- Trace minerals (including potassium, iron, magnesium, calcium, zinc)
- Vitamins (including B1, B2, B6, and D)
- Chlorophyll
- Fatty acids (including omega-3 and omega-6)
- Ketones
- Terpenes
- Flavonoids
- Glycosides
- Water
- Pigments
- Nitrogenous compounds

For more details on the essential vitamins, minerals, proteins, and healthy fats which can be found in CBD oil, check out **Plus CBD Oil** (at *pluscbdoil.com/blog.html*).

Some brands advertise their CBD as being "isolate", "full spectrum", or "broad spectrum". While none of these terms are regulated, but they can be helpful differentiators:

- **CBD isolate** usually means pure CBD, where no other cannabinoids or other naturally occurring substances like flavonoids or terpenes are present.

- **Full spectrum CBD** means everything that occurs in the hemp plant alongside the CBD, including trace amounts of THC (in most cases less than 0.3%) and other cannabinoids, such as cannabigerol and anti-oxidant compounds.

- **Broad spectrum CBD** means that it's an extract that is between full spectrum and isolate, but with no THC detectable.

So as explained, cannabis is the psychoactive variety of the plant, which is used to alter states of consciousness. It is the illegal substance. **Hemp is the legal, non-psychoactive variety**, which is useful for medicine and many other products.

THE SCIENCE BEHIND IT

There have been a lot of scientific tests into the benefits of hemp and CBD oil to see what impact it can have on the human body, to see just how effective it can be to help with ailments. This chapter will take a look at the most important ones to give you a deeper understanding.

NationalGeographic.com has presented **a range of studies that have been conducted over time:**

- *The Chemist.* In 1963, Raphael Mechoulam, a young, organic chemist, worked for the Weizmann Institute of Science outside Tel Aviv, Israel, and conducted a study. He tested it on monkeys to see the calming effects on them. He discovered some positive changes in neuroprotection, movement, balance, memory, and immune health.

- *The Botanist.* Phillip Hague, a horticulturist who believes CBD has displayed some promise, at least, anecdotal, in the treatment of disorders and diseases, such as amyotrophic lateral sclerosis, osteoporosis, psoriasis, dementia, schizophrenia, multiple sclerosis, and post-traumatic stress disorder.

- *The Biochemist.* Manuel Guzmán is a lead scientist in working with mice to shrink their tumors using CBD. He's been very successful so far with the animals.

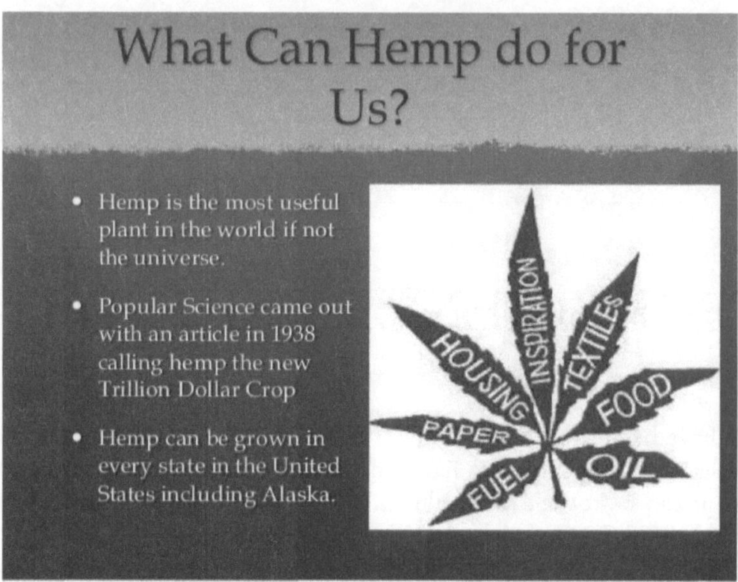

The **Journal of Neuropsychopharmacology** and **Medical and Biological Research** have presented reports on the **calming effects CBD has on the brain.** Even the **World Health Organization** has confirmed this. It **produces therapeutic and neuroprotective effects**, which is **because of the following:**

- *Serotonin Receptors.* A Brazilian study (at *ncbi.nlm.nih.gov/pubmed/24923339*) has found that CBD activates an inhibitory response in the 5-HT1A serotonin receptor, which is implicated in processes such as anxiety, appetite, addiction, pain perception, nausea, sleep, and vomiting.

- *Neuroprotective Effect.* Researchers (at *ncbi.nlm.nih.gov/pubmed/18679164*) discovered that CBD reduces short-term brain damage by increasing oxygen to the brain.

- *TRPV-1.* It helps calm down the pain receptors in the brain.

It also **has effects on the body,** as shown by the study presented at **Equities** (at *equities.com/news/the-science-of-cbd*):

- It activates the 5-HT1A receptor, which prevents nausea.

- It binds TRPV-1 receptors, which moderate pain and body temperature.

- It blocks G protein receptor GPR55, which decreases bone reabsorption and the spreading of cancer cells.

- It activates peroxisome proliferator-activated receptors, which help fight cancer and Alzheimer's.

A study presented at **High Times** (at _hightimes.com/health/cbd/the-biology-of-cbd/_) shows that while CBD has similar biological effects to THC, the changes in behavior are the complete opposite.

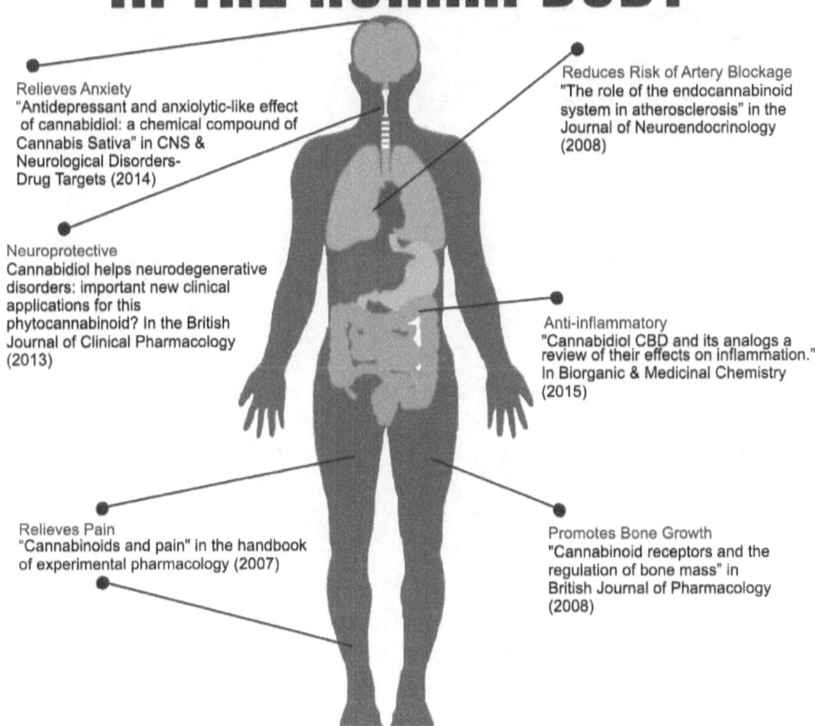

There are always more studies being conducted and new research coming out, which gives a much bigger insight into the benefits of CBD oil, deepening our understanding.

The Endocannabinoid System

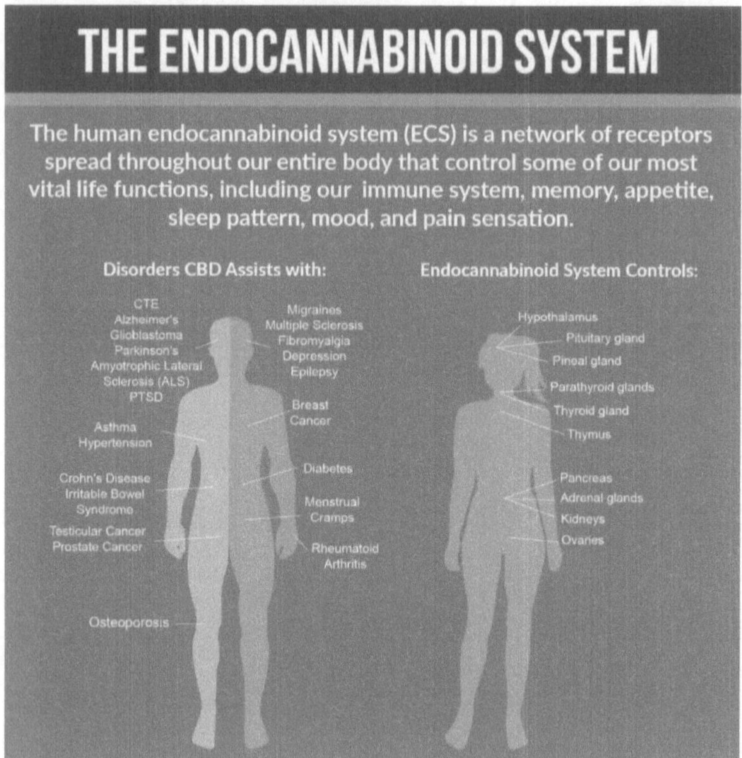

The Endocannabinoid System (or **ECS**) is the biological system that binds cannabinoid receptors, making the effects of the CBD more effective. **These particular cell receptors** are the body's natural THC. They **can regulate:**

- Sleep patterns
- Digestive system
- Mental stability
- Body control
- Immune system
- Fertility
- Pain and nerve damage
- Memory loss
- Temperature

The endocannabinoid system consists of cannabinoid 1 (CB1), which the receptors are found in the brain and nervous system, and cannabinoid 2

(CB2), which is found in the immune system. This gives it control over the majority of functions in the body.

If this is low, CBD oil can help restore it and bring you back to your natural self. It replaces anything you may be missing to get those functions back in top form. It doesn't bind the receptors, like traditional medicine; it works alongside it to **boost the body's natural ability to take care of itself**.

There is a big debate into whether **alternative medicine or traditional medicine** is better, which, of course, this comes into. There are many arguments for both, but if you'd like to read more into the scientific research behind it, try these studies:

- Complementary and Alternative Healthcare: Is It Evidence-Based? (*ncbi.nlm.nih.gov/pmc/articles/PMC3068720/*)

- Mysticism and/or rigor: Can science and alternative medicine shake hands? (*columbia.edu/cu/21stC/issue-3.4/walker.html*)

- Complementary and alternative drug therapy versus science-oriented medicine (*ncbi.nlm.nih.gov/pmc/articles/PMC4480118/*)

	Conventional Medicine	*Alternative Medicine*
Mind, Body & Spirit	Separate entity	Unified one
Consider Human as	A machine	Microcosm (universe)
Disease due to	Infection/organ defect	System imbalance
Role of Medicine	Fight infection/combat disease by suppressing symptoms	Restore harmony, which make their symptoms disappear
Treatment Focus	Matters – parts/organs	Energy – holistic (whole)
Treatments	Correct the part/organ	Promote self-healing
Primary Interventions	Drugs, surgery	Diet, exercise, herbal medicine & manipulation
Treatment Purpose	Just sick care	Total health care

10 SURPRISING FACTS ABOUT HEMP

You might think you already know everything there is to know about hemp and CBD, but this chapter will probably give you something new to think about.

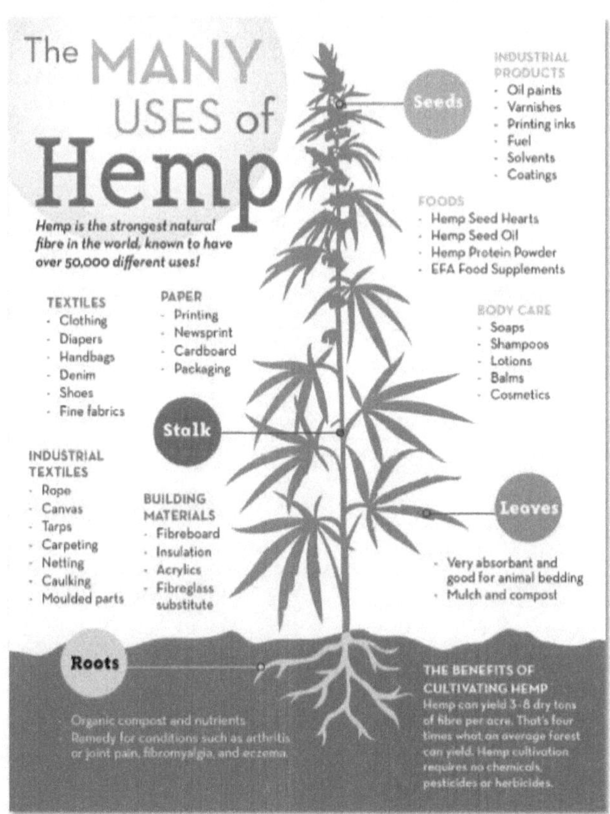

1. It's impossible to overdose on CBD since it's nontoxic.

2. CBD is actually safe for use in pets suffering from health conditions such as arthritis/joint pain, epilepsy, skin problems, and anxiety.

3. The royal family have actually used CBD. One notable example is that of Queen Victoria, who ruled England from 1837 to her death in 1901.

4. Hemp can actually help the environment because it eliminates toxins and radiation from the environment. So much so, scientists discovered hemp extracted more chemicals from surrounding soil, due to phytoremediation, than other plants in Chernobyl.

5. CBD has created a culture of medical tourism, as people desperately travel to places where they can acquire it legally to cure a selection of ailments, because it's the only thing they think will help them.

6. Rather than getting users 'high,' CBD can actually reduce the effects of THC, particularly the negative side effects.

7. It never shows up on drugs tests…because it isn't a drug.

8. CBD oil is a must have in the beauty bag because it has amazing effects on your hair and skin.

9. In 2003, the US Patent office has recognized CBD as an antioxidant.

10. Hemp seeds have more nutrition than flax or chia. They are classified as a superfood.

	Protein	Omega-6	Omega-3	GLA	SDA	Carbs
Hemp Hearts	10.0g	8.0g	2.5g	384mg	128mg	3.0g
Flax	5.6g	0	4.5g	N/A	N/A	9.6g
Chia	6.3g	1.8g	6.3g	N/A	N/A	12.3g

Per 30g or 3 tbsp
*average of three different sources/brands

Source: ManitobaHarvest.com

TOP 8 HEALTH BENEFITS OF CBD

There are many benefits to using CBD as already shown, but this chapter will provide the top eight for you to consider. These will be examined in much more detail later on in the book, so if there's something in particular that interests or affects you, then you'll be able to find it.

1. Pain

There have been studies (at _ncbi.nlm.nih.gov/pmc/articles/PMC2503660_) into the dulling effects it has on pain. By interrupting the messages from the brain to the body, the user doesn't feel the pain as acutely. Not surprisingly, according to _Gallup_ data roughly four out of ten men and women who use CBD products, say they use them for pain relief.

2. Appearance

Scientists have also looked into the positive effects that CBD oil can have on a user's hair and body. Particularly skin disorders, due to the CBD working with the endocannabinoids in the body.

3. Heart

Heart disease and the positive effects that CBD can have on it have also been looked into. The CB1 receptors are blocked, calming the valves down.

4. Mental Health

Researchers agree that by calming the nerves down, CBD can have a very positive effect on mental health suffers. By working with the body's natural serotonin, it boosts users up.

5. Hormones

CBD also works very well to balance the hormones that have become imbalanced. A study (at _ncbi.nlm.nih.gov/pubmed/8257923_) into the effect it can have on cortisol shows this.

6. *Immune System*

The CBD's combination with the endocannabinoid system in the body boosts the immune system to help combat viruses and bacteria.

7. *Joints*

For illnesses such as arthritis, CBD can really help with the stiffness and pain in the joints. Particularly if these issues are degenerative, because of the boosted immune system.

8. *Nervous System*

Because CBD can calm down the nerves inside the body, it produces several actions driven by its neuroprotective, anticonvulsive, anti-inflammatory, sedative, antipsychotic, and hypnotic properties.

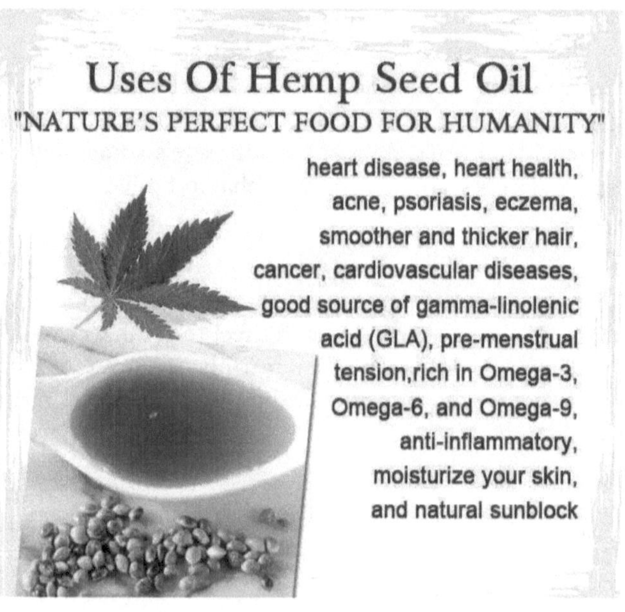

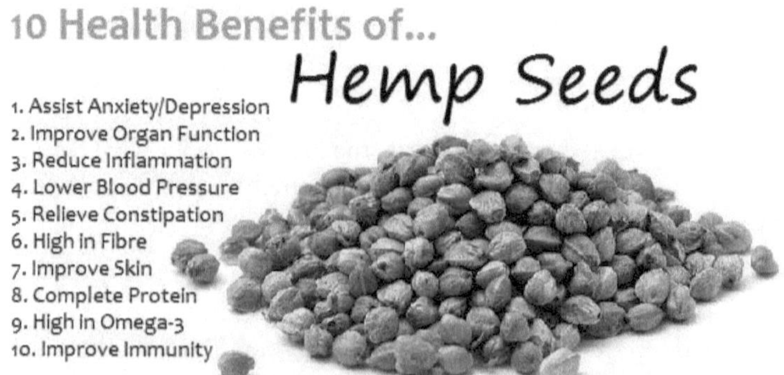

THE MOST COMMON AND UNIQUE WAYS TO USE CBD

There are **a few ways to take CBD**, and if it's your first time, this can feel a little overwhelming. This chapter is a guide to help you with this, but you can always ask a medical professional if you would like some help.

1. *Swallow and Ingest*

The most common way, and the recommended way for best results, to take the oil is to swallow pure oil. This way it can pass through your digestive system and get metabolized by the liver. Active compounds will then be delivered into your bloodstream. Most CBD oils come with an easy-to-use applicator to make this process very simple.

2. *Held Under the Tongue*

It's also common to hold the oil under the tongue so the mucus membranes in the mouth can absorb the active compounds for the fastest delivery. It also provided he highest levels of bioavailability Again, you can use the syringe-like applicator to put the oil under your tongue. Simply place the correct quantity of drops under your tongue using the dropper and hold the CBD oil in place between 1 and 2 minutes for it to absorb.

3. *Cooking*

Many people like to include CBD seamlessly into their everyday lives so it isn't so much of a life change, making it easier to remember. It's easy to add to smoothies, acai bowls, coffee, salads, oatmeal, ice cream, and curries. Just remember that CBD oil tends to evaporate at temperatures higher than 160-180°C, or 320-356°F.

4. *Topical*

You can apply CBD to your skin in a cream form, or even as a shampoo or shower gel. There are many products on the market for you to try.

5. *Capsule*

You can also get capsules if you cannot take the oil in any other form. These are just like tablets and are very easy to take.

6. *Vaporize*

Vaping has become very popular in the recent years because it doesn't affect lungs in a negative way. The fumes are absorbed into the bloodstream. Their bioavailability is rather low because half of product gets blown out. The vaping pens are easy to buy from any local store. Vape pens *must not* be the kind made for nicotine as it's too hot and burns the CBD.

7. *Gum*

You can even buy gum, which contains 50 mg of non-GMO hemp oil and 10 mg of CBD. (*medicalmarijuanainc.com/can-chew/*)

TIP:

Do not take CBD oil at the same time as when you take your other pharmaceuticals, wait at least few hours.

The recommended dosage for each of these methods is unique, depending on the condition being treated and who you are. The *Cannabidiol Dosage Guide* (at *projectcbd.org/guidance/cannabis-dosing*) suggests that you should consult a health practitioner first to get some advice and always begin with a low dosage, then work your way up if need be. Overdoing it can create unnecessary problems. While you cannot overdose on it, taking too much can aggravate side effects.

Condition	Person Size 2-25 lbs	Person Size 26-45 lbs	Person Size 46-85 lbs	Person Size 86-150 lbs	Person Size 151-240 lbs	Person Size 240+ lbs
Mild Range	4.5 mg	6 mg	9 mg	12 mg	18 mg	22.5 mg
Mid-Range	6 mg	9 mg	12 mg	15 mg	22.5 mg	30 mg
Severe Range	9 mg	12 mg	15 mg	18 mg	27 mg	45 mg

10 SAFETY TIPS THAT YOU SHOULD KNOW

While CBD has got many benefits, you do need to make sure that you use it carefully, so here are the **top 10 safety tips to help you** with this:

1. Always **get advice from a medical professional**, especially if you have previous health conditions, before using CBD oil to get the best guidance that's personal to you. Everyone is different and has individual needs, so it's always best to be certain. Liver issues can be particularly tricky.

2. Learn about **the potential side effects** so you know what to look out for. While this oil is nontoxic, it can still have effects, such as:

   - Light-headedness

   - Drowsiness

   - Dry mouth

   - Blood pressure fluctuations

   - Heart rate issues

   - Temperature fluctuations

   - Glucose and pH level fluctuations

   - Potassium and sodium level fluctuations

3. You'll also want to be sure that it doesn't mix with any of the drugs you're currently taking. Here is **a list of ones to be careful with:**

   - Anesthetics

   - Angiotensin II blockers

   - Antibiotics

   - Antihistamines

- Anti-arrhythmics
- Anti-depressants
- Anti-epileptics
- Anti-psychotics
- Benzodiazepines
- Beta blockers
- Calcium channel blockers
- HIV antivirals
- HMG CoA reductase inhibitors
- Immune modulators
- NSAIDs
- Oral hypoglycemic agents
- Prokinetics
- PPIs
- Steroids
- Sulfonylureas

4. You need to **store the oils right**. In an upright position at a stable temperature and away from extreme light, heat, or moisture. It's best to store in a cupboard, but some people do keep it in the fridge between uses.

5. **Check those 'Best Before' dates**. They are important! Unopened, it lasts 14 months (*hempoil.ca/shelf-life-of-hemp-oil*); opened, it's 6 months.

6. While **pregnancy** often brings with it pain, nausea, and stress, it's advisable to keep away from CBD during this time because there aren't enough studies to guarantee its safety. When pregnant, always get advice from a doctor before taking anything.

7. The same goes for **breastfeeding**. It's advisable to stay away from CBD oil when it comes to feeding your young child, but if this is something you want to do, then consult a medical professional first.

8. When it comes to **children**, there is a lot of conflicting advice and opinions. Some parents swear by it, especially if their children suffer from an affliction such as epilepsy. It's best to seek medical advice first. Many researchers suggest it's not for children under 10 years old (*cbdschool.com/is-cbd-hemp-oil-safe/*).

9. While you cannot overdose, always **follow the guidelines** of what is recommended for you to take for optimum results. Some of the factors to take into account when using CBD are your medical condition, the severity of your problem, your body weight, metabolism, and sensitivity to cannabis (how you respond to CBD).

10. **Do your research**. While this book can give you a general overview, it's up to you to work out how the oil can help you as an individual with your condition and lifestyle. Don't take anything until you fully know what you're getting yourself into.

Know your types as well. Do you want medicinal hemp oil or non-medicinal essential oil? For more information on the right brands and purity for your usage, check the next chapter. You can also find out more about how to scientifically test the oil at home at *cnbs.org/drug-test-kits/marijuana-thc-test-kits.*

THE ULTIMATE GUIDE FOR BUYING CBD HEMP OIL

5 Most Common Mistakes to Avoid

Because there are so many oils out there on the market, it can feel overwhelming when you take that first step. To get the best results, you need to buy high quality, pure oil, so here are some tips to help you ensure that you're not making any of **the 5 most common mistakes**:

1. **Low prices** – because there are so many options, companies compete to have the lowest cost product out there. But this can sometimes mean that the quality isn't as high. If it's a low concentration, then you won't get the results you're looking for.

2. **A 'cure all'** – there isn't an oil that cures everything. Each one is made to treat certain ailments; so if you have a specific issue, then you need to pick a suitable one.

3. **The 'non-psychoactive' stamp** – you'll need to find one with this stamp to be sure that it's legal. Buying from a reputable seller is a great way to ensure this.

4. **Extraction method** – if an oil has been made by a licensed pharmacist, then it'll be created using the correct techniques, ensuring your product is pure. Supercritical (or subcritical) Co2, ethanol, and olive oil are the extraction methods to look for. Note that Butane extraction is cheap and efficient but toxic to make and use, so you should try to avoid companies using this extraction method.

5. **Reviews** – check the company details before you buy, other customers' opinions are very important.

Little-Known Tips to Choose the Best Quality Oil

The factors to look out for to see if you're buying high quality oil is:

- *Quality* – if the product is a 'whole plant' extract, then the quality will be higher.

- *Quantity* – you'll be able to get a varying size pot of CBD oil. If it's your first time, go for the smaller size to confirm it suits you. Some companies even offer samples.

- *Price* – the price can be anything from a couple of dollars to over $100. It's best to take a look at all the other factors, plus the reviews, to confirm you're getting what you want.

- *Cannabidiol Strength* – an ideal strength will be 450-900 mg. Make sure that the ingredient list states "cannabidiol". For first time users it's recommended to start with a minimum of 240 mg+ in a 10ml bottle.

- *Purity* – it shouldn't be over 80%, otherwise it'll be too high. Ask the brand or check to see if they provide evidence of third-party certification on the purity and stated amount of the CBD.

- *Organic* – the word 'organic' doesn't necessarily mean the product is all natural. Check the ingredients first ensuring they are certified organic and wildcrafted. A label indicating that a product is "USDA Organic" or "Certified Organic" means that at least 95% of the ingredients are obtained from organic sources.

- *Packaging* – the packaging is very important, because it'll help make the product last longer. Cardboard boxes and glass bottles are best.

- *Bioavailability* – 250 mg of CBD should contain 250 mg of actual active CBD.

- *THC Content* – confirm it is less than 0.3%.

- *Sourcing* – hemp needs to be grown outdoors in the right climate. Mild, humid, and with 20 to 30 inches of rain per year.

- *Third-party test results* – these tests can tell you about the product including the cannabinoid content and if it contains any potential dangerous materials.

- *Absorption* – you want the absorption of the oil to be over 6%.

Don't forget: if you're struggling to find out any of these things, you can just ask. If buying in store, ask the person who works there, and if purchasing online, send an email first. You can ask about where the oil is sourced, how it's reviewed, the strength and purity, etc., but if you want something more personalized to your health condition, it might be better to check with a medical professional who will understand your condition better.

What is the Legal Status of CBD Oil?

The legality of the oil is something else that might concern you, so here is a guide to help you. This lets you know where you can buy the oil and where you might have trouble. Again, for the most up to date information, consult a medical professional who will be able to help you with the best advice, including how to legally acquire it.

The distinction between hemp and marijuana means that **any CBD product made from hemp that contains less than 0.3% THC is legal under federal law in the United States.**

You can buy CBD products online, or in-store throughout the United States without a prescription.

Legal Status of CBD in the United States

State	Hemp-Derived	Marijuana-Derived	By Prescription	Legislation
Alabama	Legal	Illegal	Legal	Allowed only for epilepsy cases (Carl's Law 2014)
Alaska	Legal	Legal	Legal	
Arizona	Legal	Illegal	Legal	
Arkansas	Legal	Illegal	Legal	
California	Legal	Legal	Legal	
Colorado	Legal	Legal	Legal	
Connecticut	Legal	Illegal	Legal	
Delaware	Legal	Illegal	Legal	Allowed only for chronic epilepsy and muscle contractions (Rylie's Law 2015)
Florida	Legal	Illegal	Legal	Allowed for approved special cases with no more than 8% THC (2014)
Georgia	Legal	Illegal	Legal	Allowed only for extreme conditions such as Sclerosis with no more than 5% THC (Haleigh's Hope Act 2015)
Hawaii	Legal	Illegal	Legal	
Idaho	Legal	Illegal	Illegal	
Illinois	Legal	Illegal	Legal	
Indiana	Legal	Illegal	Legal	Allowed only for chronic epilepsy with no more than 0.3% THC (2017)
Iowa	Legal	Illegal	Legal	Allowed for chronic Sclerosis conditions with no more than 3% THC (2017)
Kansas	Legal	Illegal	Illegal	
Kentucky	Legal	Illegal	Legal	Allowed only for approved cases of epilepsy (2014)
Louisiana	Legal	Illegal	Legal	Allowed for chronic Sclerosis conditions (2016)

Maine	Legal	Legal	Legal	
Maryland	Legal	Illegal	Legal	
Massachusetts	Legal	Legal	Legal	
Michigan	Legal	Illegal	Legal	
Minnesota	Legal	Illegal	Legal	
Mississippi	Legal	Illegal	Legal	Allowed only to treat severe seizures in children with no more than 0.5% THC (Harper Grace Law 2014)
Missouri	Legal	Illegal	Legal	Allowed only for chronic epilepsy with no more than 0.3% THC (2014)
Montana	Legal	Illegal	Legal	
Nebraska	Legal	Illegal	Illegal	
Nevada	Legal	Legal	Legal	
New Hampshire	Legal	Illegal	Legal	
New Jersey	Legal	Illegal	Legal	
New Mexico	Legal	Illegal	Legal	
New York	Legal	Illegal	Legal	
North Carolina	Legal	Illegal	Legal	Allowed only for chronic epilepsy with no more than 0.3% THC (2014)
North Dakota	Legal	Illegal	Legal	
Ohio	Legal	Illegal	Legal	
Oklahoma	Legal	Illegal	Legal	Allowed only for chronic epilepsy with no more than 0.3% THC (2015)
Oregon	Legal	Legal	Legal	
Pennsylvania	Legal	Illegal	Legal	
Rhode Island	Legal	Illegal	Legal	
South Carolina	Legal	Illegal	Legal	Allowed only for chronic epilepsy with no more than 0.9% THC (Julian's Law 2017)
South Dakota	Legal	Illegal	Illegal	
Tennessee	Legal	Illegal	Legal	
Texas	Legal	Illegal	Legal	Allowed only for chronic epilepsy with no more than 0.9%

				THC (Charlee's Law 2015)
Utah	Legal	Illegal	Legal	
Vermont	Legal	Illegal	Legal	
Virginia	Legal	Illegal	Legal	Allowed only for chronic epilepsy with no more than 5% THC (2014)
Washington	Legal	Legal	Legal	
West Virginia	Legal	Illegal	Legal	
Wisconsin	Legal	Illegal	Legal	Allowed only for special conditions (2017)
Wyoming	Legal	Illegal	Legal	Allowed only for chronic epilepsy with no more than 0.3% THC (2015)

Legal Status of CBD Around the World

State/Country	CBD Legal Status	Hemp Cultivation Legal Status	THC Legal Status	THC Legal Limit in Hemp Oils
Argentina	Medical Only	Hemp Legal	Banned	0.2%
Australia	Medical Only	Hemp Legal	Banned	Not Listed
Austria	Medical Only	Hemp Legal	Banned	0.3%
Belgium	Medical Only	Hemp Legal	Banned	0.2%
Belize	Medical Only	Hemp Legal	Grey-Area	Not Listed
Brazil	Medical Only	Hemp Not Legal	Banned	Not Listed
Bulgaria	Unrestricted	Hemp Legal	Banned	0.2%
Canada	Unrestricted	Hemp & Marijuana Legal	Unrestricted	Not Listed
Chile	Medical Only	Hemp & Marijuana Legal	Medical Only	Not Listed
China	Unrestricted	Hemp Legal	Banned	0.3%
Colombia	Unrestricted	Hemp & Marijuana Legal	Unrestricted	1%
Costa Rica	Grey Area	Hemp Not Legal	Grey-Area	0.5%
Croatia	Medical Only	Hemp Legal	Banned	0.2%
Cyprus	Medical Only	Hemp Legal	Banned	0.2%
Denmark	Unrestricted	Hemp Legal	Banned	0.2%
Estonia	Unrestricted	Hemp Legal	Banned	0.2%
Finland	Grey Area	Hemp Not Legal	Banned	Not Listed
France	Unrestricted	Hemp Legal	Banned	0.2%
Georgia	Grey Area	Hemp Not Legal	Banned	Not Listed
Germany	Unrestricted	Hemp Legal	Banned	0.2%
Greece	Unrestricted	Hemp Legal	Banned	0.2%
Guatemala	Banned	Hemp Not Legal	Banned	Not Listed
Hong Kong	Grey Area	Hemp Legal	Banned	0%
Hungary	Unrestricted	Hemp Legal	Banned	0.2%
Iceland	Grey Area	Hemp Legal	Banned	0%
India	Grey Area	Hemp Legal	Banned	Not Listed
Ireland	Unrestricted	Hemp Legal	Banned	0.2%

Israel	Medical Only	Hemp Legal	Grey-Area	Not Listed
Italy	Grey Area	Hemp Legal	Banned	0.2%
Japan	Unrestricted	Hemp Legal	Banned	0%
Latvia	Unrestricted	Hemp Legal	Banned	0.2%
Lithuania	Unrestricted	Hemp Legal	Medical Only	Not Listed
Luxembourg	Unrestricted	Hemp Legal	Grey-Area	0.3%
Malta	Medical Only	Hemp Legal	Medical Only	Not Listed
Mexico	Grey Area	Hemp Not Legal	Restricted	1%
Netherlands	Unrestricted	Hemp & Marijuana Legal	Grey-Area	0.05%
New Zealand	Medical Only	Hemp Legal	Banned	2%
Norway	Unrestricted	Hemp Not Legal	Banned	0%
Paraguay	Unrestricted	Hemp Legal	Restricted	Not Listed
Peru	Medical Only	Hemp Legal	Medical Only	1%
Poland	Unrestricted	Hemp Legal	Banned	0.2%
Portugal	Medical Only	Hemp Legal	Medical Only	0.2%
Puerto Rico	Unrestricted	Hemp Legal	Medical Only	0.3%
Romania	Unrestricted	Hemp Legal	Banned	0.2%
Russia	Grey Area	Hemp Legal	Banned	0.2%
Singapore	Banned	Hemp Not Legal	Banned	0%
Slovakia	Banned	Hemp Not Legal	Banned	0%
Slovenia	Unrestricted	Hemp Legal	Unrestricted	0.2%
South Africa	Restricted	Hemp Legal	Banned	Not Listed
South Korea	Medical Only	Hemp Legal	Banned	0%
Spain	Unrestricted	Hemp Legal	Grey-Area	0.2%
Sweden	Unrestricted	Hemp Legal	Banned	0%
Switzerland	Unrestricted	Hemp Legal	Banned	1%
Turkey	Medical Only	Hemp Legal	Banned	0.2%
United Kingdom	Unrestricted	Hemp Legal	Banned	0.2%
United States	Unrestricted	Hemp Legal	Grey-Area	0.3%
Uruguay	Unrestricted	Hemp & Marijuana Legal	Unrestricted	1%
Virgin Islands	Medical Only	Hemp Legal	Medical Only	0.3%

Top 10 Trusted CBD Oil Brands

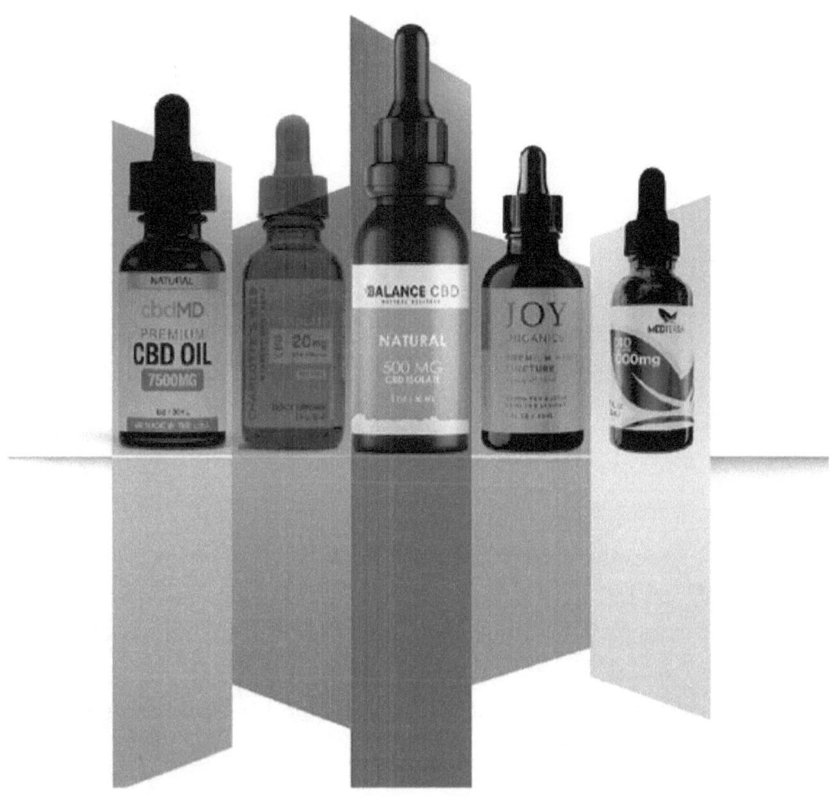

Below are some of the **most recognized CBD oil brands**.

Kanibi

kanibi.com

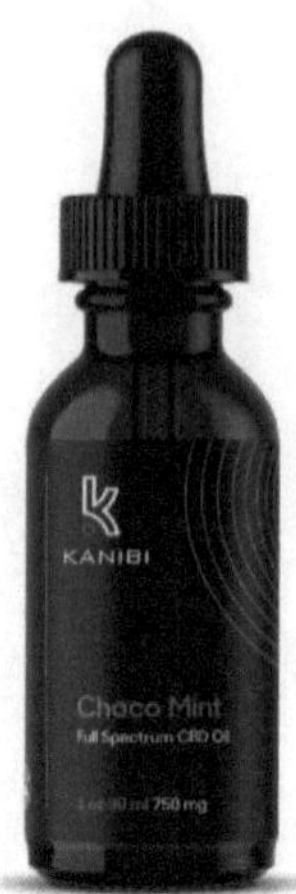

- One of the best CBD manufacturers of highest quality products

- A huge product range including oils, creams, gummies, and soft gels

- Great tasting products that are double lab-tested for strict quality control

cbdMD

cbdmd.com

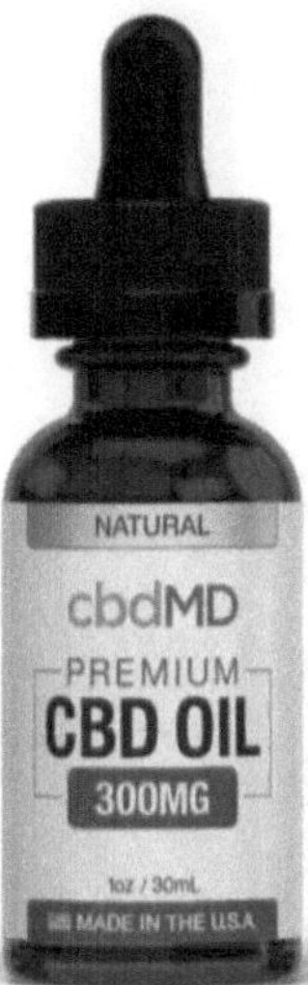

- Truly high-quality products for an affordable price

- Broad-spectrum CBD oils in variety of strengths and flavors

- Uses a base of MCT oil and offers some of the most powerful dosages on the market

- Third-party test results from SC labs

PureKana

purekana.com

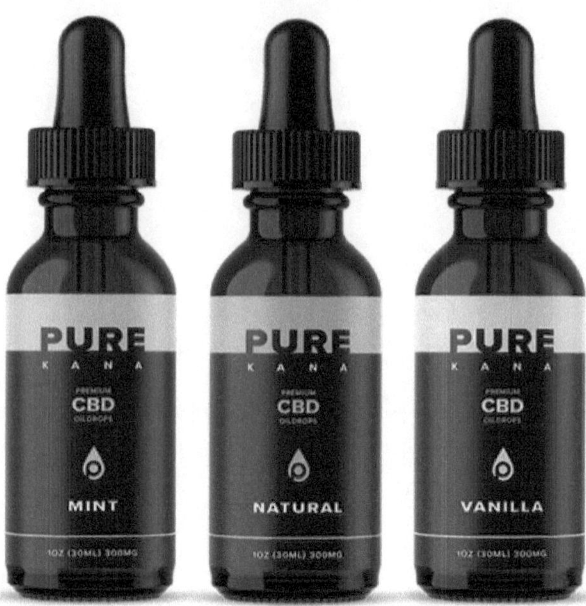

- 100% organic and non-GMO products

- One of the top CBD oil producers of 2017 using the most advanced CO2 extractions methods

- Lab-tested to produce 99% product purity and also provides tests by third-party labs

NuLeaf Naturals

nuleafnaturals.com

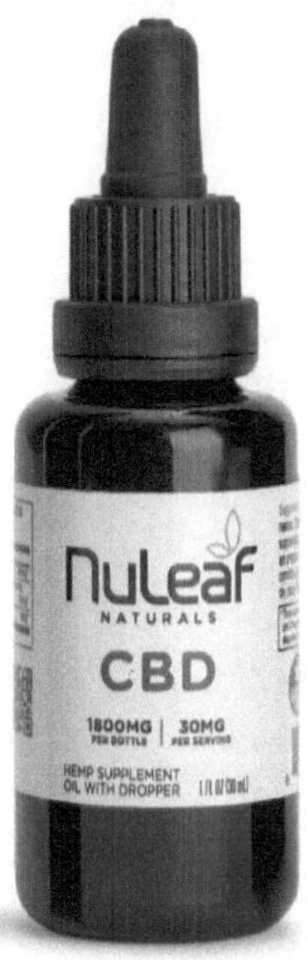

- Highest quality products that are free from toxins, chemicals, flavors and additives

- CBD oils only contain only two ingredients: USDA-certified organic hemp seed oil and full spectrum hemp extract

- Each product delivers 50 mg of full spectrum CBD per 1 mL of oil

- Cost of CBD per mg starts from $0.09

- Provides third-party lab reports

Fab CBD

fabcbd.com

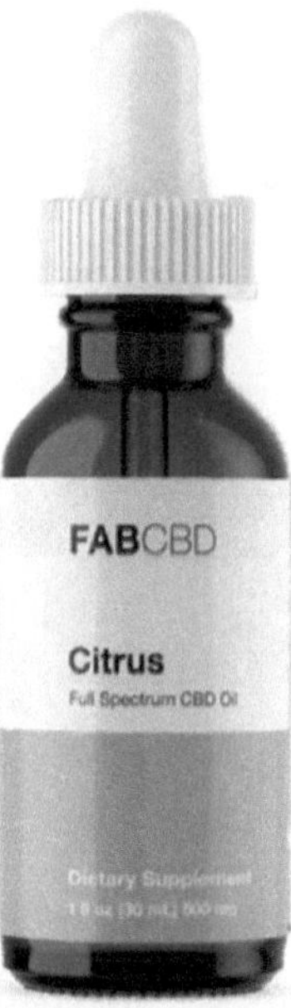

- Full spectrum non-GMO CBD oils sourced from organically grown hemp in Colorado

- Oils are made to order and they are paired with fractioned coconut oil

- Comes in five all-natural flavors in strengths of 300 mg, 600 mg, 1200 mg and 2400 mg per bottle

- Cost of CBD per mg starts from $0.09

- Third-party lab testing reports are available

- CBD dog treats, topical cream and best-rated CBD gummies

Joy Organics

joyorganics.com

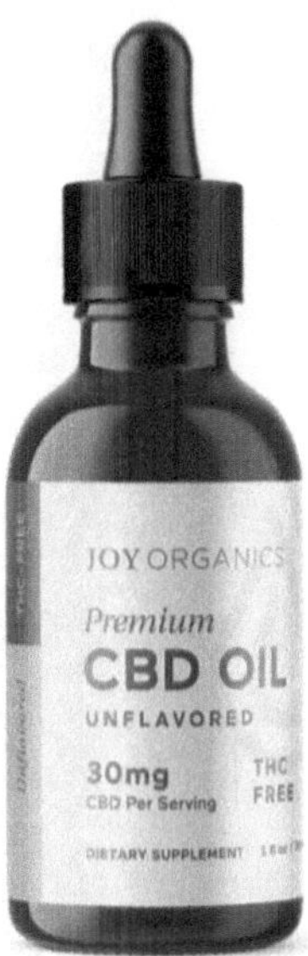

- THC-free broad-spectrum products using proprietary hemp strains organically grown in the USD

- Extracted with organic extra-virgin olive oil, providing a base that makes for a smooth intake

- Comes in four flavors in dosages of 7.5 mg to 15 mg per serving

- Cost of CBD per mg starts from $0.07

- Third-party lab testing reports

Spruce

takespruce.com

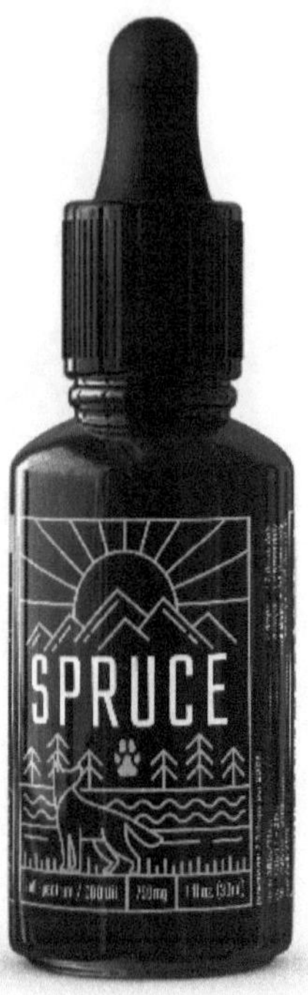

- Some of the highest potency, full spectrum oils derived from organic hemp farms in the USA

- Focuses on small-batch CBD production, helping to ensure consistency and quality of the products

- Comes in two strengths - 25 mg or 80 mg per serving

- Cost of CBD per mg starts from $0.11

- Third-party lab testing reports from ProVerde Laboratories are available

CBDistillery

thecbdistillery.com

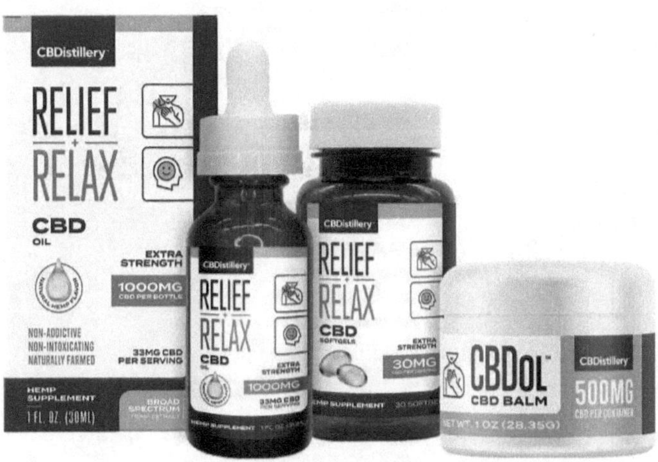

- Products are US Hemp Authority certified

- Derived from organic non-GMO and pesticide-free industrial hemp farms in the USA

- Wide variety of product options including oils, creams, vapes, capsules, soft-gels, and gummies

- Cost of CBD per mg starts from $0.06

- 88% of their customers reported that CBD helped with mild or temporary anxiety

- Full-spectrum and THC-free tinctures with strengths ranging from 33 mg to 83 mg per serving

Balance CBD

balancecbd.com

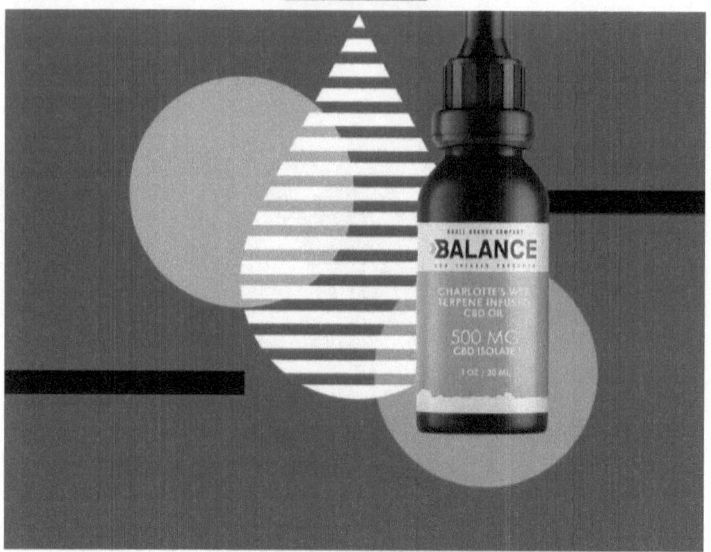

- Highest quality all-natural non-GMO organic products from US farms

- Cost of CBD per mg starts from $0.03 – one of the best value on the market

- Wide variety of product options including CBD oils for dogs, CBD creams, CBD vape pens, CBD edibles, and gummies

- Third-party lab testing reports are available on their website

Elixinol

elixinol.com

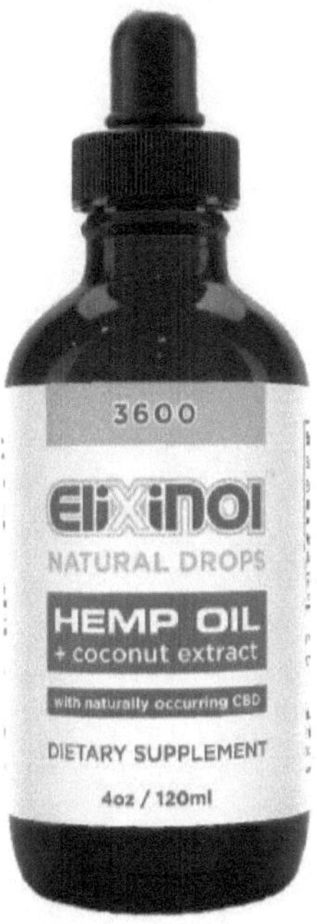

- Massive variety of products

- World-renowned CBD vendor having received multiple media recognitions

- Product prices range from $39 to $250

Also look out for other brands such as **PremiumJane** (at *premiumjane.com*), **MedTerra** (at *medterracbd.com*), **CW Botanicals** (at *charlottesweb.com*), or **Pure CDB vapors** (at *purecbdvapors.com*), to name just a few.

50 LITTLE-KNOWN USES FOR CBD

As you have seen so far in this book, there are many **positive uses for CBD oil** to improve your health. This chapter will go into more detail about 50 of these uses to give you more information on each.

A Special Note About Dosing

When it comes to dosing, it is all about how many milligrams (mg) of the active ingredient (CBD) are in the oil or the capsule. Pure CBD molecules need to be carried or infused in something that is a **delivery system**. If your CBD product suggest dispensing "drops", then that's a *unit of administration*. Note that most droppers dispense 30 drops for every mL of oil. If your CBD product suggest serving/administration size is 1 mL (milliliter), then 1 mL is the *unit of administration*.

According to *CBDOilReview.org* the **serving standard** of CBD oil is 25 mg taken twice daily.

As a general **cautious approach**:

- take 10 – 15 mg of CBD per day for 2-3 days. The CBD improves as it builds up in your system. If you feel much better, stay with that dose. A daily dose between 0.5 and 20 mg is considered a microdose for most of the common ailments.

- If you need to feel more relief, then take 20 – 30 mg of CBD per day for 2 – 3 days. If you feel much better, stay with that dose. Be consistent and patient. You should feel some results, but in some cases, it can take a week or two to gauge your improvement.

- After 6 -7 days if you still want to feel better, increase the dose to 50 mg per day. Stay with that for 1 week. In some cases, 50 mg in the morning can be good followed by 20 – 50 mg at night. CBD stays in the system for about 12 hours.

For a more **substantial approach**:

- Take 25 mg of CBD per day for 2 days. This is NOT an aggressive dose at all. A standard dose of CBD is considered 10 to 100 mg per day for most conditions.

- If you need to feel more relief, then take 50 mg of CBD per day for 2 days. If you feel much better, stay with that dose. CBD is clinically shown to be safe with almost no side effects (until doses of 600 – 1,000 mg/day are administered).

- After 4 – 5 days if you still want to feel better, increase the dose to 50 to 100 mg per day. Stay with that for 1 week. In some cases, 50 – 75 mg in the morning can be good followed by 50 – 75 mg at night. If you are trying to reduce a migraine headache, you'll need to take 150 mg in one dose.

When it comes to cannabis therapy, often times "less is more", so if you're not getting the desired results from a higher dose, then you should consider lowering your dose instead of increasing it.

For more information about CBD oil dosage guidelines, please check *Hemppedia.org*.

1. *Constant Pain*

Constant, often referred to as chronic, pain is defined as *"any pain lasting more than 12 weeks. Whereas acute pain is a normal sensation that alerts us to possible injury, chronic pain is very different. Chronic pain persists—often for months or even longer."*

Chronic pain can result from a single injury but doesn't subside when it should. As well as limited flexibility and pain, this can lead to other issues such as mood swings, fatigue, decreased appetite, and sleep disturbances.

CBD oil can help with the pain itself, the associated inflammation, and any other discomfort, and is safer than habit-forming medications like opioids. The chemicals in the oil react with the brain receptors and immune system, giving a similar pain-killing effect. Studies have confirmed this, many times (e.g. *healthline.com/health/cbd-oil-for-pain#chronic-pain-relief*).

TIP: To instantly relieve pain on an open wound (cuticles, skate board scrapes, etc.) or on a canker sore (in the mouth), use one drop of CBD liquid tincture.

Dosage: Over the course of 25 days, begin with 2.5-20 mg of CBD daily by mouth, then revise according to your needs (increase if you need more).

Application: Oil or capsules.

Precautions: You will need to consult a medical professional first to ensure it will work with any other medications you're taking. Side effects can include tiredness, diarrhea, and appetite changes.

2. *Fibromyalgia*

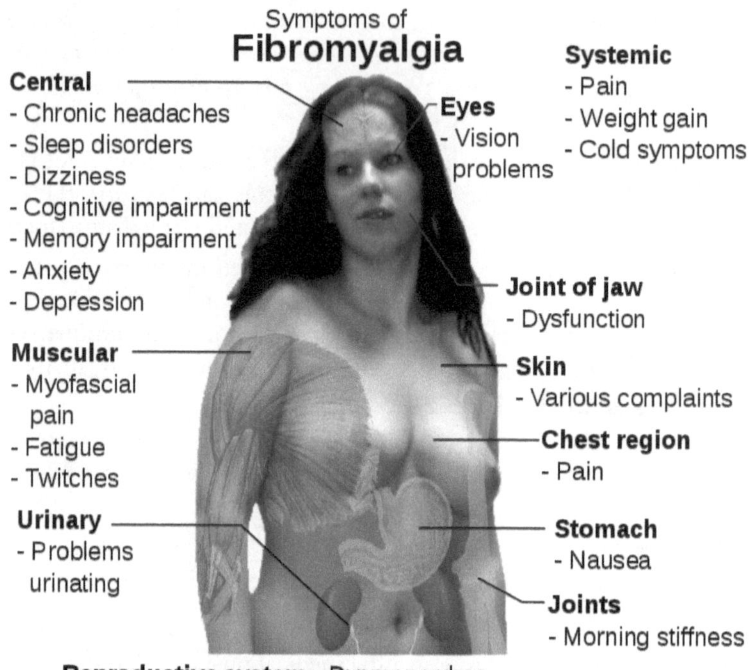

Fibromyalgia is a chronic condition causing pain throughout the body. Symptoms include heightened sensitivity to pain, muscle stiffness, fatigue, headaches, difficulty sleeping, concentration and memory issues, and irritable bowel syndrome.

This condition's cause could be related to an abnormal level of chemicals in the brain that change the nervous system and how pain messages are carried throughout the body, but is technically unknown. This can occur during stressful events, such as giving birth, having an operation, or even emotional stress.

Many fibromyalgia sufferers have found their symptoms were reduced when using CBD oil. The pain, spasms, and stiffness are alleviated as the CBD calms down the nervous system.

Dosage: Over the course of 25 days, begin with 2.5-20 mg of CBD daily by mouth, then revise according to your needs (increase if you need more).

Application: Oil, capsules, or vape. If you decide to use a vape, make sure to only use *low-heat* vapes to avoid ingesting/inhaling burned carcinogens.

Precautions: Be aware of the side effects of CBD because it may make any dizziness worse. These can include dizziness, nausea, dry mouth, and drowsiness.

3.   *Autoimmune Disorders*

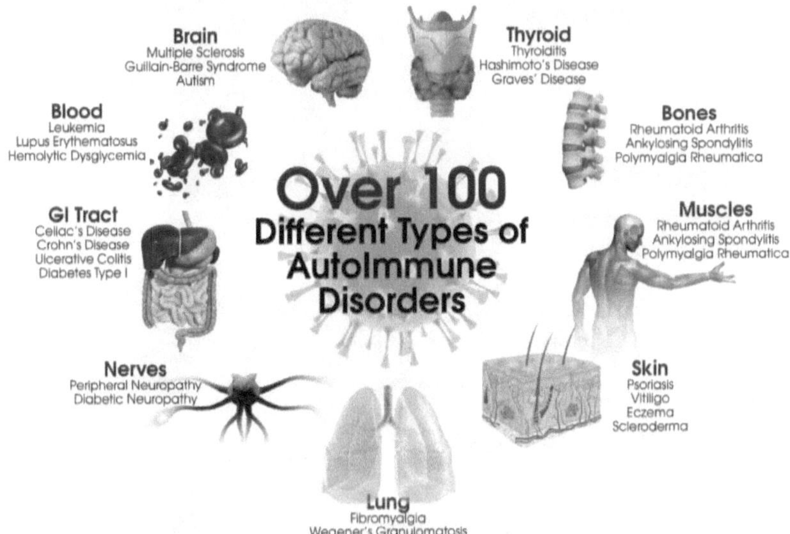

Autoimmune disorders are conditions in which your immune system mistakenly attacks your body. Your immune system protects your body from germs, bacteria, and viruses, but if you suffer from one of these conditions, your body does this to normal cells, attacking them because it thinks they shouldn't be there. Lupus, vasculitis, and Celiac disease are just a few of these illnesses.

Anyone suffering from these illnesses can have their whole body affected by pain, muscle issues, nerve problems, and skin issues – all of which CBD works to calm down. It is suggested that the oil gives a sense of stability, a mood elevation, and a reshaping of the body structure, all of which helps people live better with these diseases.

Dosage: This is dependent on your specific condition. Consult a medical professional first.

Application: Oil or capsules.

Precautions: Check with a doctor regarding your current medicine list. One of the potential side effects of CBD is making the body take longer to absorb other medication, so you'll need to be certain of this information before you start using CBD.

4. *Rheumatoid Arthritis*

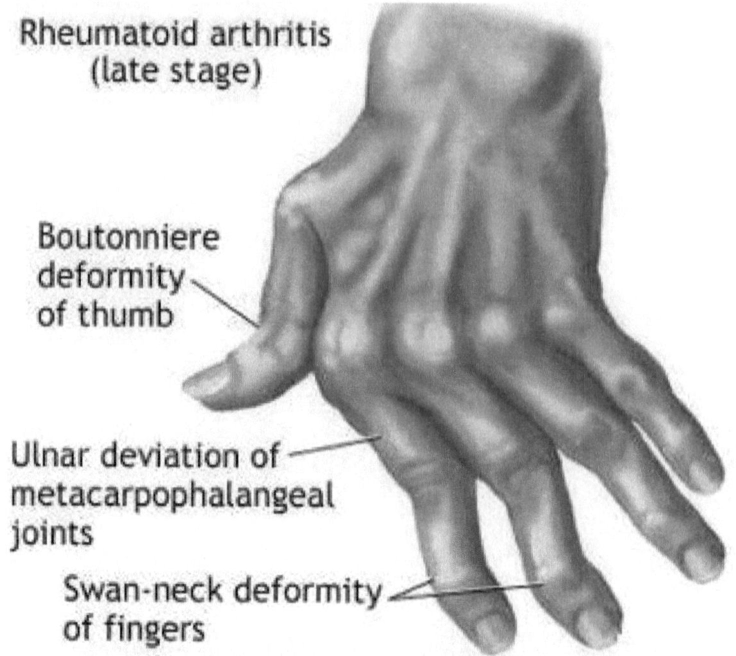

Rheumatoid arthritis is a long-term condition that causes pain, swelling and stiffness in the joints. The symptoms usually affect the hands, feet and wrists. There are many flare-up periods with this condition that makes the pain much worse. The people who are most likely to be affected by this are women who smoke with a family history of the illness.

Studies conducted found that long-term use of CBD helped with the joint pain and swelling significantly (e.g. *healthline.com/health/cbd-oil-for-rheumatoid-arthritis*). The oil stops your immune system from attacking your joints.

Dosage: Start with 2.5 mg three times a day and increase if needed.

Application: Oil, capsule, or topically applied to the affected area.

TIP: For arthritis or joint pain, you can achieve faster results by using a CBD pain cream alongside your CBD oil (e.g. *royalcbd.com/product/cbd-cream*).

Precautions: Speak to a medical professional about your condition and current medication list first. Side effects can include tiredness, trouble sleeping, feeling irritable, and nausea.

5.   *Muscle Spasms*

Muscle spasms are most common and are often due to overuse and muscle fatigue, dehydration, and electrolyte abnormalities. The spasm occurs abruptly, is painful, and is usually short-lived.

This is usually a short-term problem, but if it becomes a greater issue, you should speak to a doctor about the potential cause. Possible causes are issues with your discs or spine. These can be dangerous.

Because this is an issue with the nervous system, CBD can have a very positive effect on your body, easing some of the strain. Many researchers have looked into this.

Did you know that while it varies on a person to person, but it takes around 20-40 minutes for the body to react to CBD after it's taken?

Dosage: You will want to check out the chart below and start with the lowest daily dosage, increasing it if necessary:

Condition Range	Size Person 31-60 lbs	Size Person 61-100 lbs	Size Person 100-175 lbs	Size Person 175-250 lbs +
Mild 1	2mg-4mg +	4mg-6mg +	6mg-8mg +	8mg-10mg +
2	4mg-8mg +	6mg-12mg +	8mg-18mg +	12mg-20mg +
Medium 3	8mg-12mg +	12mg-18mg +	18mg-24mg +	22mg-30mg +
4	12mg-18mg +	18mg-24mg +	24mg-32mg +	32mg-40mg +
Severe 5	18mg-30mg +	24mg-40mg +	32mg-60mg +	42mg-60mg +

Application: Oil, capsules, or applied topically to affected area.

Precautions: Check with your trusted medical professional. You want to learn the underlying cause. Side effects can include stiffness, dizziness, and sickness.

6. *Migraines*

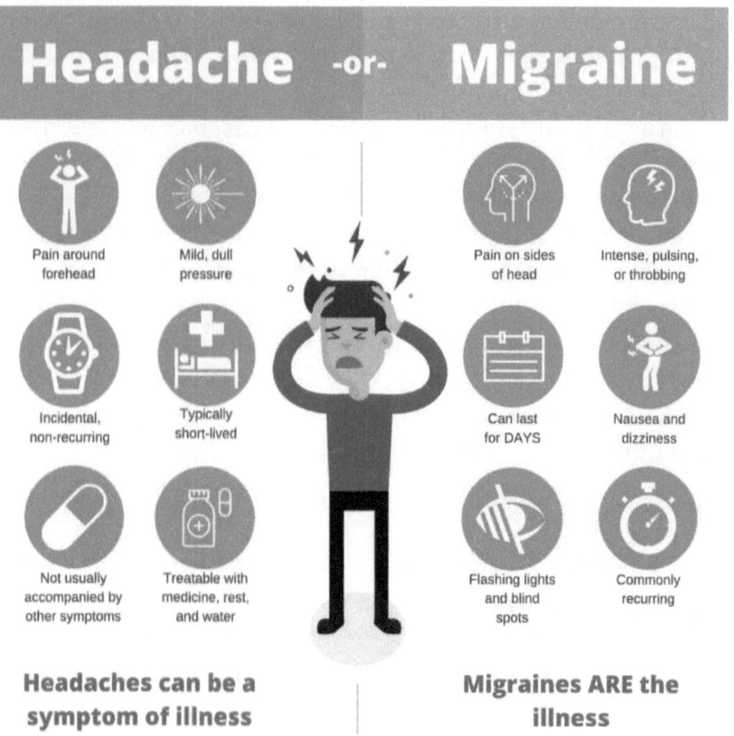

Migraines are a severe form of headache that usually brings with it sensitivity, nausea, and vomiting. It affects one in five women and one in fifteen men. This is a challenging, but fairly common, disorder than can be treated with painkillers (although, not too many!). But if it's accompanied with paralysis or weakness, slurred speech, blinding pain, or a high temperature, then it's time to seek a medical intervention.

A 2017 study found that using CBD oil gave a better quality of life to migraine suffers, with some having fewer migraines overall (e.g. *healthline.com/health/migraine/cbd-oil-for-migraines*). Again, this is achieved by calming down the nervous system.

Dosage: 20-25 mg of oil per day (e.g. *idweeds.com/cbd-migraines*).

Application: Oil or capsules.

Precautions: Be aware of the side effects, in particular dizziness.

7. *Multiple Sclerosis*

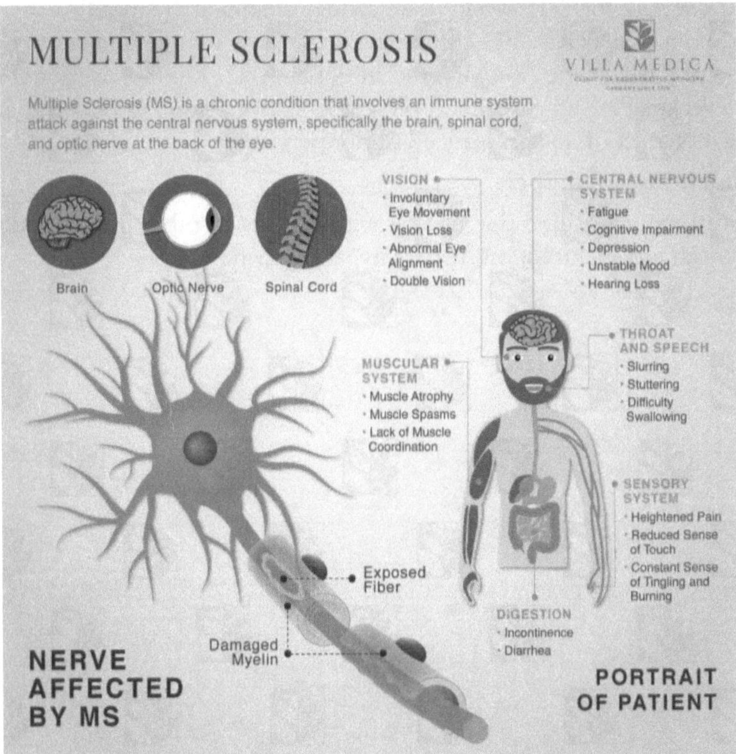

Multiple sclerosis is a condition that affects your spinal cord and brain, causing eye problems, arm and leg movement issues, and balance struggles. This is a lifelong condition that can range from mild all the way to severely disabled.

Main symptoms are:

- Bladder problems

- Blurred vision

- Fatigue

- Issues with planning, learning, and thinking

- Numbness or tingling

- Problems with balance

- Spasms and muscle stiffness

- Struggling with walking

CBD cannot cure the disease, but it can help with the symptoms by working with the nervous system, reducing neuropathic pain, spasticity, muscle spasms, and sleep disturbances.

Dosage: Daily for 2-15 weeks, take cannabis extracts by mouth containing 2.5-120 mg of a THC-CBD combination. A single mouth spray can contain 2.5 mg of CBD and 2.7 mg of THC in doses of 2.5-120 mg, use for at most eight weeks. Patients usually apply eight sprays within three-hour increments, at a max of 48 sprays in a 24-hour period.

Application: Mouth spray.

Precautions: Consult a doctor first with regards to other medication. Side effects can include tiredness, irritability, and dizziness.

8.   *Spinal Cord Injuries*

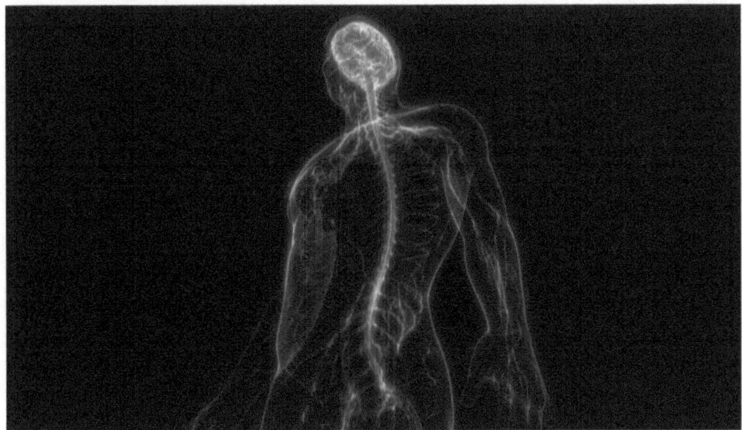

Spinal cord injuries can be very dangerous because they often cause changes in strength, sensation, and body functions. You must always consult a medical professional if you think you might have one, because there may be immediate treatment that you need to ensure the damage doesn't worsen or become permanent.

Symptoms include:

- Balance difficulties
- Bowel and bladder control issues
- Changes in libido/sexual desire
- Difficulties with circulatory system
- Inability to feel cold or heat
- Neck or back pain
- Numbness or tingling
- Pain or nerve damage
- Spasms
- Struggles with movement
- Twisted back or neck
- Weakness in the body

Several studies have already confirmed the ability of CBD to treat symptoms of spinal cord injury including spasticity, pain, depression, and insomnia. CBD has also been used effectively to treat bowel and bladder problems. Generally, the medicinal properties of CBD make it an amazing therapeutic aid for this condition.

Dosage: Start with 25 mg per day and increase if needed.

Application: Oil, capsules, or topically applied to the affected area.

Precautions: Be aware of the side effects. These can include tiredness or inability to sleep, fatigue, and changes to appetite.

9. Inflammation

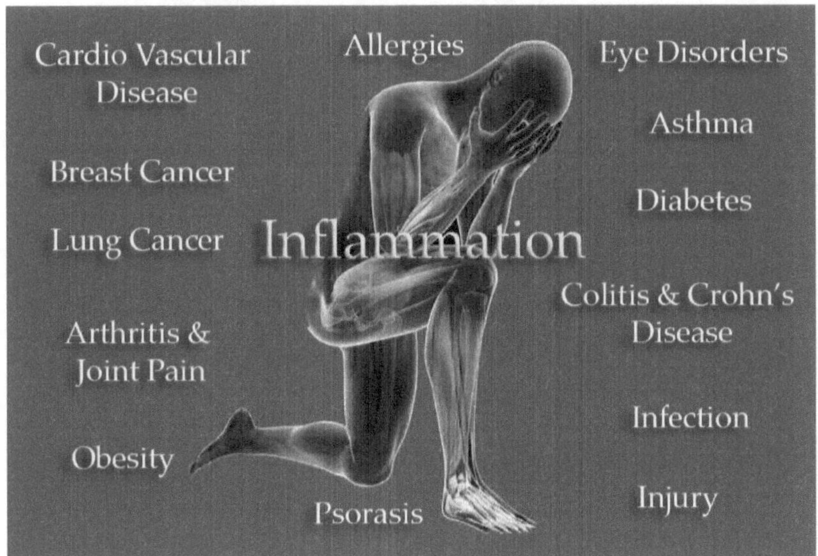

Inflammation is one of your body's defense mechanisms employed while the body heals. It's a very useful process, which the body must go through in order to recover. If it lasts longer than necessary, this is when you might want to get it looked at.

The symptoms of acute inflammation are as follows:

- *Pain*: An inflamed area can feel painful to the touch. Chemicals are released, which stimulate nerve endings and make that area feel more sensitive.

- *Redness*: This is due to capillaries in that area being filled with more blood than normal.

- *Immobility*: Inflammation may cause some loss of muscle or body function in that region.

- *Swelling*: This is typically caused by fluid buildup.

- *Heat*: This is caused by more blood flow to the inflamed area.

CBD works with the body's endocannabinoid system to have a therapeutic reaction.

Dosage: 2.5-20 mg of CBD by mouth daily.

Application: Oil or capsules.

Precautions: Consult a doctor to learn the source of the inflammation first. Side effects can include dry mouth, fatigue, and nausea.

10. Seizures

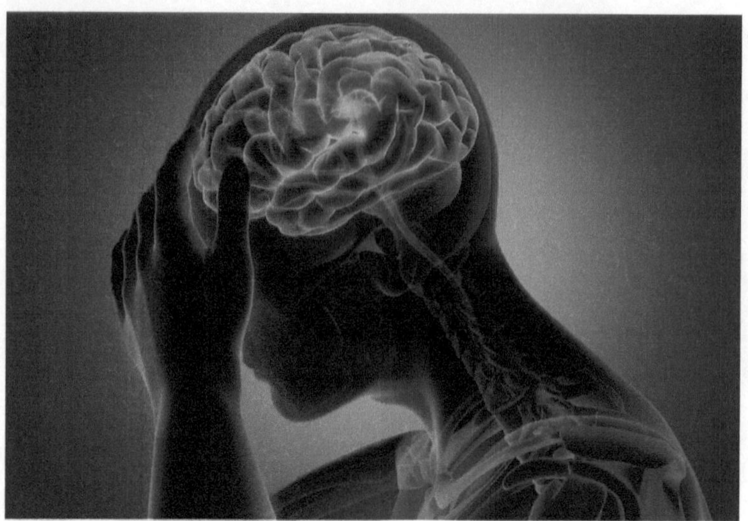

Seizures are symptoms of a brain problem. They happen because of sudden, abnormal electrical activity in the brain. They are not always convulsions, though, and can last from 30 seconds to 2 minutes. If they last longer than 5 minutes, this may be a larger medical emergency.

Epilepsy is the most well-known cause of seizures and is defined in the dictionary as *"a neurological disorder marked by sudden recurrent episodes of sensory disturbance, loss of consciousness, or convulsions, associated with abnormal electrical activity in the brain."*.

Did you know that each year, about 150,000 Americans are diagnosed with epilepsy?

Many studies have agreed that CBD can calm down, and in some cases reduce the number of, seizures as it works well with the nervous system.

Dosage: Apply 200-300 mg of CBD daily by mouth. You can also use online forum at *epilepsy.com/connect/forums/medication-issues/cbd-dosage* for more information.

Application: Oil or capsule.

Precautions: Speak to a medical professional about the side effects and your current medication. Side effects may include sleepiness, diarrhea, fatigue, and decreased appetite.

11. Schizophrenia

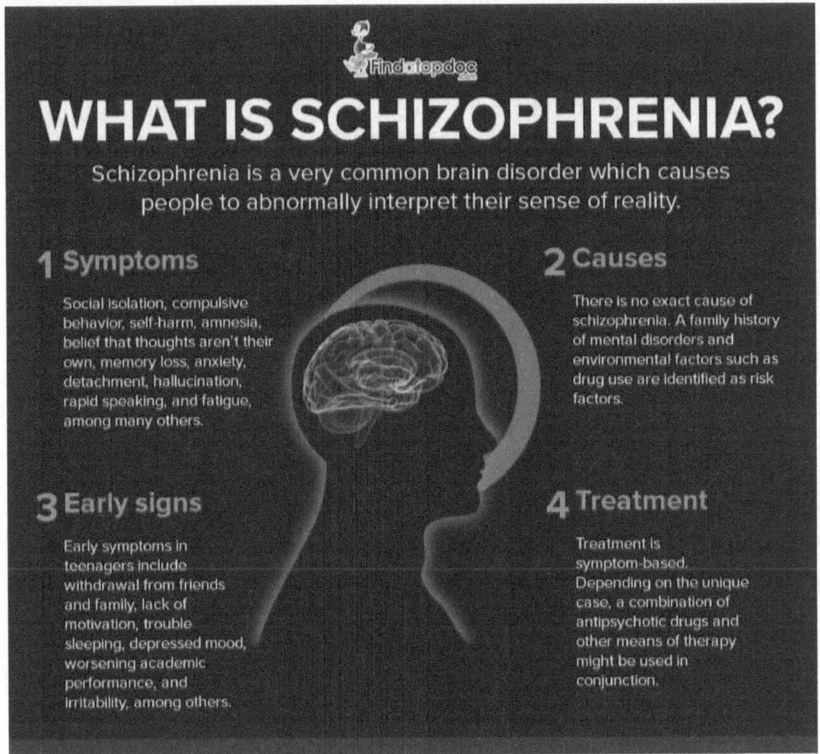

Schizophrenia is a mental disorder characterized by abnormal social behavior and failure to understand reality. Common symptoms include false beliefs, unclear or confused thinking, hearing voices that others do not, reduced social engagement and emotional expression, and a lack of motivation.

The symptoms of this are listed as:

- A lack of interest in the world around you
- Feelings of disconnect
- Struggles with concentrating
- Wanting to be alone
- Hallucinations
- Delusions
- A struggle to organize thoughts and speech
- Disinterest in yourself

It leaves sufferers unable to cope with day-to-day activities because confusion and suspicion get in the way. If this is something you suspect you might have, a medical intervention is necessary before the symptoms get worse.

CBD has been studied with regards to schizophrenia, along with other psychological disorders, and it's been found by T.A. Iseger and M.G. Bossong in 2015 (at *ncbi.nlm.nih.gov/pubmed/25667194*) that: *"The first small-scale clinical studies with CBD treatment of patients with psychotic symptoms further confirm the potential of CBD as an effective, safe and well-tolerated antipsychotic compound."*

It may not be able to cure the problem, but it can reduce many of the symptoms.

Dosage: Apply 40-1,280 mg CBD daily by mouth, dependent on weight and severity of condition.

TIP: For bipolar or schizophrenia, larger doses work better. 125 – 150 mg per dose may help stabilize mood, and going up to 600 mg dose may address actual mania.

Application: Oil, capsule, or vape.

Precautions: Don't make changes to your current medical plan without speaking to a doctor first. Side effects can include blockage of your current medications, sleeplessness, restlessness, and digestive issues.

12. Autism

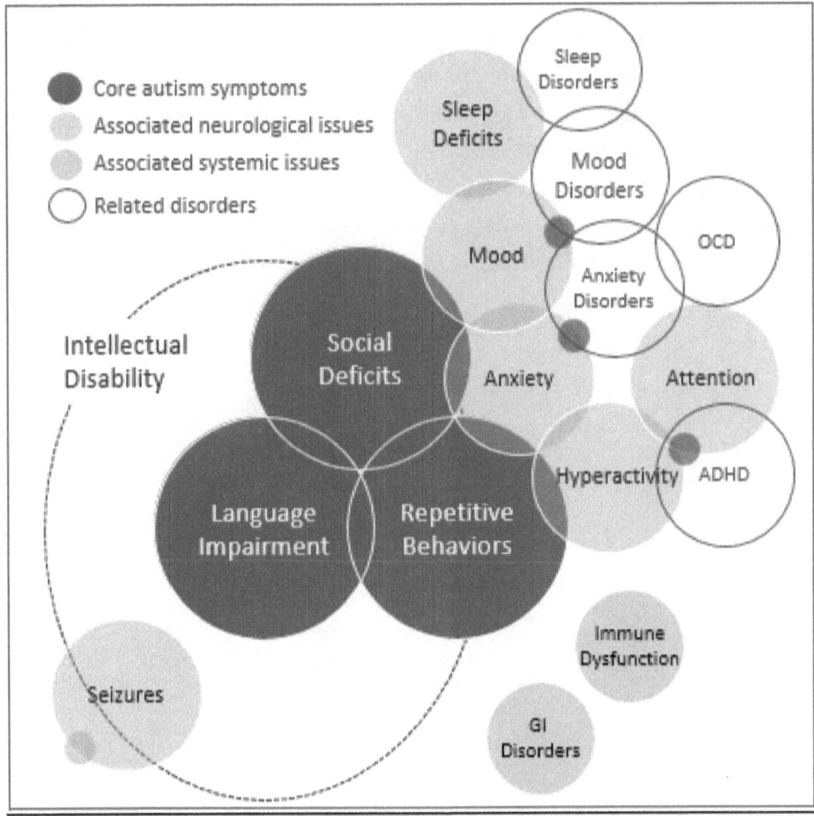

Autism is a lifelong developmental disability that affects how people perceive the world and interact with others. Suffers view and see the world differently to everyone else, but also from one another. No sufferer is exactly the same.

People who suffer from this do not comprehend tone of voice, facial expressions, and jokes or sarcasm as well as others, which means they may come across as insensitive, overwhelmed or act in a socially inappropriate way. The best way to get individual help for this is from a medical professional.

Where there isn't much official data into the testing of cannabis-based products and autism, there is one notable study (at _leafly.com/news/health/how-does-cannabis-consumption-affect-autism_) in particular by Dr. Giovanni Martinez, who is a clinical psychologist from Puerto Rico. He found in his tests that: _"initially the child would become so frustrated with his inability to communicate, he would act out and injure himself. But, now that he can express himself, he laughs and enjoys life. It's incredible to see a child go from being non-_

communicative to achieving a significant improvement in quality of life – for both the child and his family.”

CBD oil cannot cure autism, but it can assist with the symptoms by working alongside the endocannabinoid system.

Dosage: Start with 25 mg taken twice a day (*idweeds.com/cbd-autism-treatment/*). Increase if needed.

Application: Oil or capsules.

Precautions: Speak to a medical professional first with regards to your current healthcare plan. Side effects can include insomnia, dizziness, and digestive issues.

13. *Irritable Bowel Syndrome*

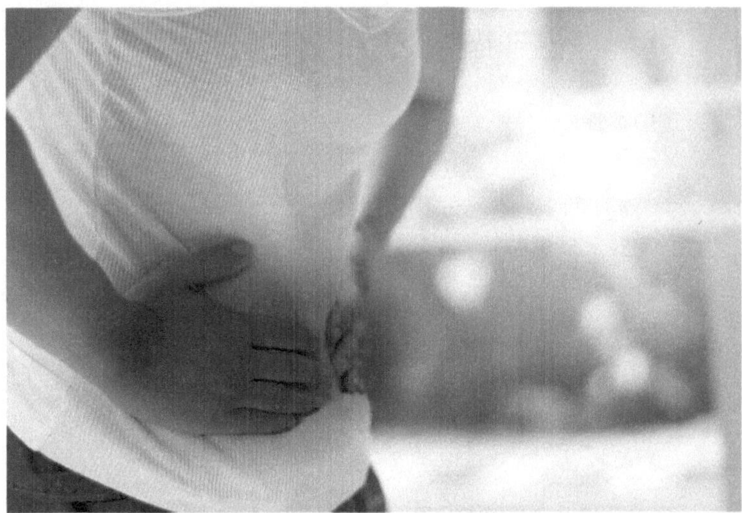

Irritable bowel syndrome (IBS) is a common disorder that affects the large intestine. Signs and symptoms include cramping, abdominal pain, bloating, gas, and diarrhea or constipation, or both. Symptoms that are a bit more severe include vomiting, weight loss, iron deficiency, nighttime diarrhea, and rectal bleeding.

IBS is triggered by certain foods, stress, or hormones. It affects twice as many women as men.

The exact cause of IBS is currently unknown, but it might be linked to the nervous system and inflammation, which, of course, CBD oil can help with. Additionally, scientists argue that CBD has analgesic and antiemetic effects. The oil will help prevent the cramping, digestive system issues, and pain.

TIP: Be cautious when taking CBD oils by mouth alongside high-fat meals. High-fat meals can dramatically increase the blood concentrations of CBD, which can increase the risk of side effects.

Dosage: Start with 25 mg twice daily and increase if needed.

Application: Oil or capsules.

Precautions: Be aware of the side effects first. They may include dizziness, diarrhea, restlessness, and fatigue.

14. Bowel Disease

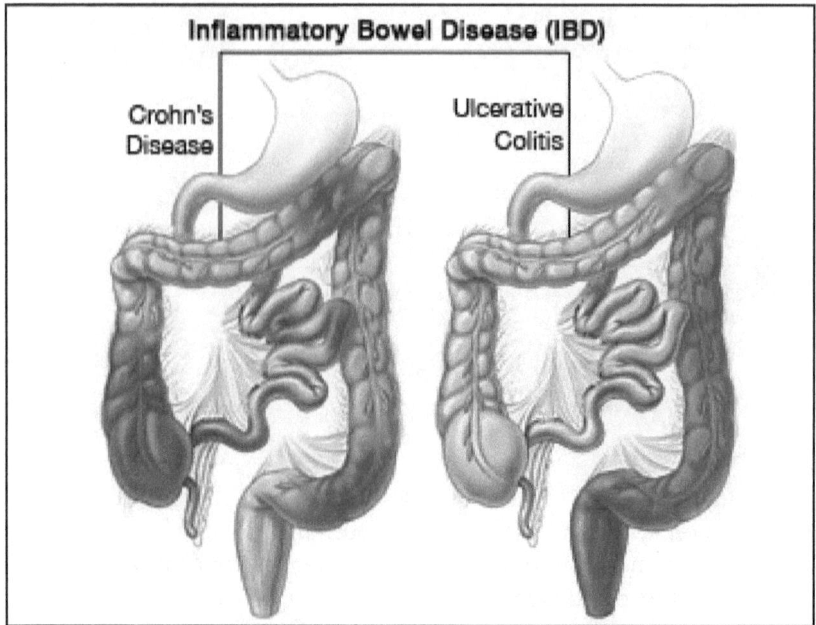

Bowel disease is an inflammation of the gut. Ulcerative colitis and Crohn's disease are specific bowel diseases that affect the colon and the entire digestive system, respectively.

Symptoms include:

- Bloody bowel movements

- Chronic fatigue

- Dramatic weight loss

- Recurring diarrhea

- Swelling of the stomach, pain, or cramps

Currently, there is no cure for IBD, only the symptoms can be cured to give sufferers a better quality of life. However, one in five people don't get any relief from traditional medication at all, which is why they are looking more and more towards alternative medication.

Studies have found that CBD oil can help ease the inflammation and pain caused by this disease (*pubmed.ncbi.nlm.nih.gov/22815234*). It also helps reduce intestinal damage, which slows down the degenerative process. There are a lot of personal stories online to give you a deeper insight as to how CBD has affected them personally, e.g. *honeycolony.com/article/cbd_crohns_disease*

Dosage: 5 mg twice daily.

Application: Oils, capsules, or vape.

Precautions: Be aware of the side effects, in particular dizziness and diarrhea.

15. Nausea

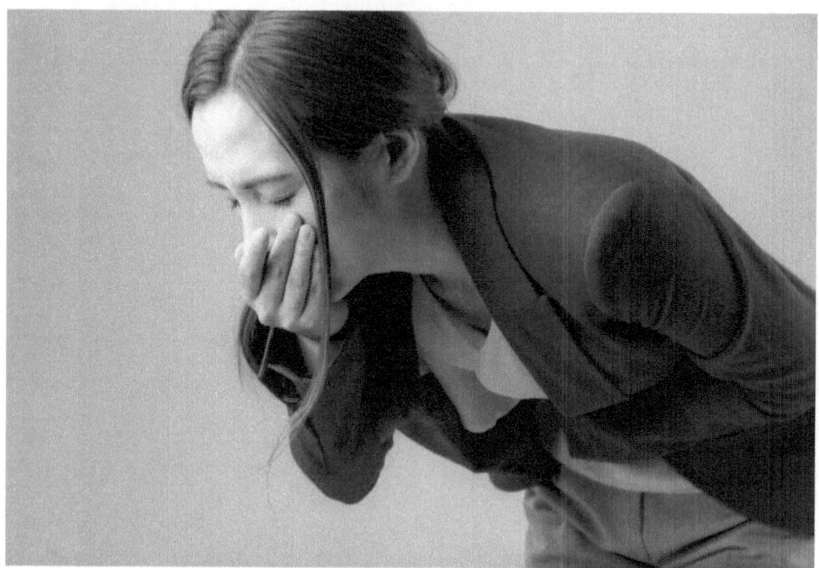

Nausea is defined as the sensation of being sick without actually vomiting, which means there may be various possible causes. A few common causes include food poisoning, motion sickness, low blood sugar, and dizziness.

According to the NHS, it is only something to really worry about, and **you'll only need to consult your doctor, if:**

- You've been vomiting repeatedly for more than 48 hours and it's not improving.

- You're unable to keep down any fluids.

- You have signs of severe dehydration – such as dizziness and passing little or no urine.

- Your vomit is green (this could mean you're bringing up bile, which suggests you may have a blockage in your bowel).

- You've lost a lot of weight since you became ill.

- You experience episodes of vomiting frequently.

Studies have found that the introduction of CBD indirectly activates a unique compound known as 5-hydroxytryptamiine-1A (5-HT1A). Through a complex biological symphony, the activation of this monoamine neurotransmitter significantly reduces the sensation of nausea and its subsequent vomiting reflex.

It's a much more natural way to alleviate the effects of nausea, whether it leads to vomiting or not. An increasing number of people are using it to reduce symptoms (although not in pregnancy, that isn't ever advised).

Dosage: 25 mg daily to start with. Increase if needed.

Application: Oil or vape.

Precautions: Be aware of the side effects, and if the symptoms persist, then you'll need a medical intervention to find the underlying cause. Side effects can include fatigue, digestive issues, and dizziness.

16. *Lack of Appetite*

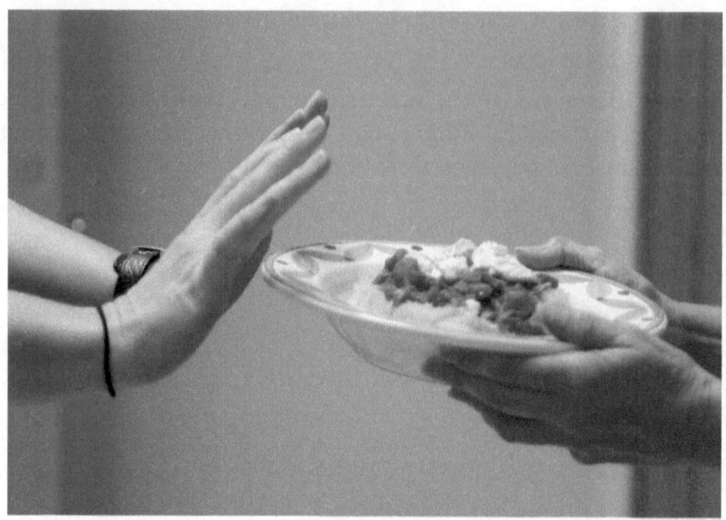

Decreased appetite is when you simply do not want to eat as much as you used to. There can be many reasons for this; it could be an underlying health issue, a psychological condition, or an effect of medication. If you don't know what's caused this, then you'll need an examination from your doctor to see what the cause could be. You should **also get checked out if any of the following occurs**:

- Racing or irregular heartbeat
- Chest pain
- Shortness of breath
- Confusion
- Dizziness
- Blurred vision
- Fainting
- Sudden weight loss
- Difficulty tolerating cold temperatures

As a neuroprotectant and antioxidant, CBD helps to calm the body's nervous system. This slows down firing signals and calms the digestive tract, helping boost appetite.

Dosage: 100-600 mg daily depending on your weight.

Application: Oil or vape.

Precautions: Be aware of the side effects, particularly low blood pressure and dizziness. If you experience any of these, speak to a doctor.

17. *Mad Cow Disease*

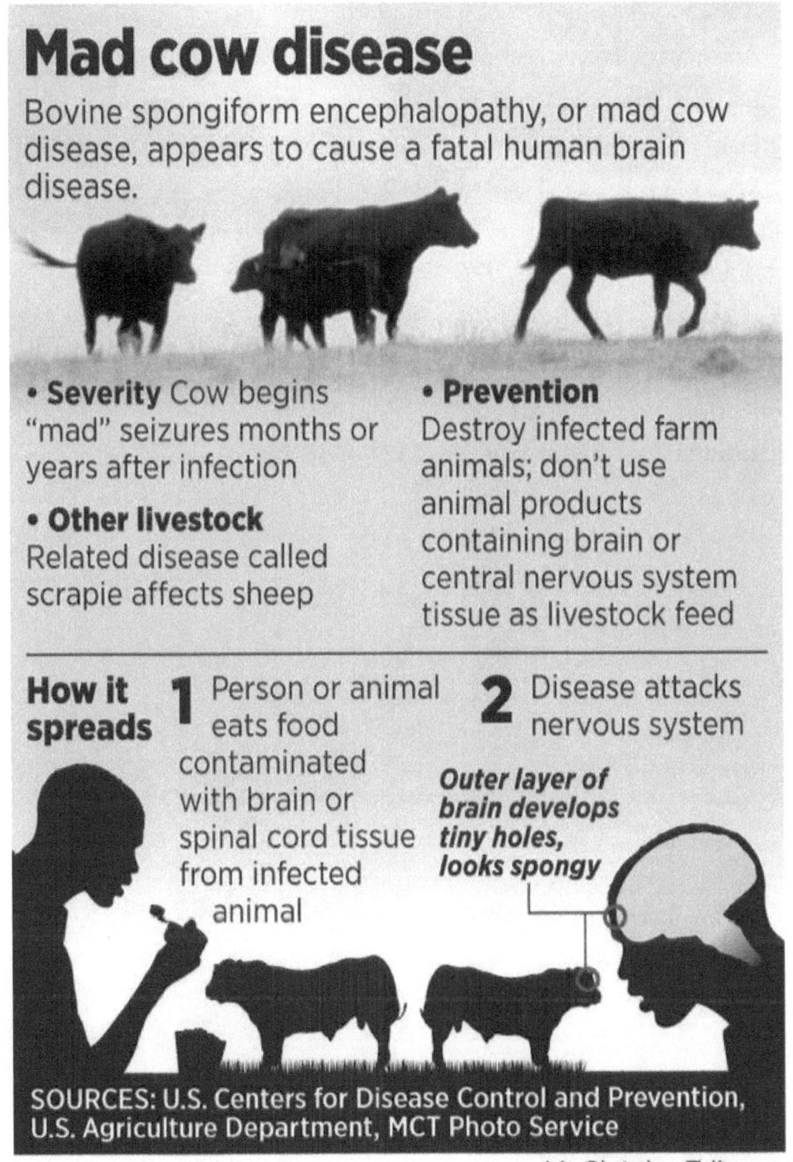

McClatchy-Tribune

Mad cow disease or bovine spongiform encephalopathy (BSE) is a transmissible spongiform encephalopathy and fatal neurodegenerative disease in cattle that may be passed to humans who have eaten infected flesh. Eating affected meat passes the disease on to humans, and it has a negative impact on the nervous system.

The **symptoms of this disease include**:

- A duration of illness of at least months
- Ataxia within weeks (or months)
- Diffusely abnormal non-diagnostic electroencephalogram
- Dementia (which displays as confusion and loss of memory)
- Myoclonus late in illness

CBD oil might not be able to cure the illness, but it can assist in alleviating the symptoms. There have been studies, but there needs to be more work into it.

Dosage: Start with 25 mg taken twice daily. Consult a doctor regarding your condition.

Application: You will need medical advice on this.

Precautions: You will need medical advice on this.

18. Alzheimer's

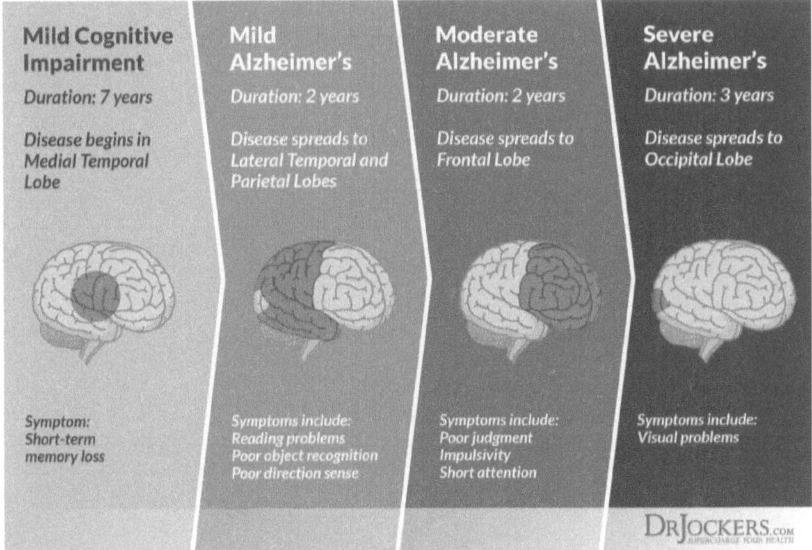

Alzheimer's disease is the most common cause of dementia. The word dementia describes a set of symptoms that can include memory loss and difficulties with thinking, problem-solving or language. The symptoms begin mild but get stronger over time. While it won't affect any two people in the same way, **here are some things to look out for**:

- Difficulties with orientation, language, concentrating, and seeing

- Forgetting about recent conversations or events

- Forgetting anniversaries or appointments

- Getting lost in a familiar place or on a familiar journey

- Losing items (such as glasses or keys) around the house

- Struggling to find the right word in a conversation or forgetting someone's name

The CBD's anti-inflammatory, antioxidant, and neurogenesis stimulant qualities can help slow the decline that Alzheimer's causes. It can also help ease the symptoms.

TIP: Don't keep taking a small dose if it's not enough to make a difference (unless it's just not affordable to go higher, in which case stick with a dose you can afford).

Dosage: You might need a medical advice on this depending on your condition, but you may start with a standard dose of 20 mg daily and increase if needed.

Application: Oil or capsules.

Precautions: Speak to a medical professional first with regards to your current healthcare plan. Side effects can include dizziness, weakness, and digestive issues.

19. *Parkinson's*

Parkinson's is a long-term degenerative disorder of the central nervous system that mainly affects the motor system. The symptoms generally come on slowly over time. Early in the disease, the most obvious are shaking, rigidity, slowness of movement, and difficulty with walking.

The symptoms to look out for include:

- Difficulty with movement
- Impaired balance
- Limb tremors
- Loss of automatic movements

- Rigid muscles

- Struggle with posture

- Slower speech

- Unable to use hands or write like they did before

It can be caused by genes, the presence of Lewy bodies (which is a protein in the brain), or environmental factors – although, this is much less likely.

An in-depth study (at *projectcbd.org/medicine/cbd-and-parkinsons-disease*) has been conducted into the usefulness of CBD and Parkinson's. The **main findings** are:

- The endocannabinoid system has a large role within Parkinson's.

- Parkinson's is associated with motor-control impairment after a critical region of the brain loses 60-80% of dopamine-producing neurons.

- Parkinson's, and the severity of its symptoms, may be affected by digestive imbalance.

- Cannabinoids might be beneficial in managing Parkinson's symptoms due to their anti-inflammatory, neuroprotectant, and antioxidant properties.

- Parkinson's symptoms may be alleviated by various combinations of THCV, THC, and CBD.

Dosage: Start with 2-5 mg of CBD oil twice or thrice daily and increase if needed. Some studies (e.g. *ncbi.nlm.nih.gov/pmc/articles/PMC5958190*) recommend taking 75 mg to 300 mg CBD oil per day.

Application: Oil or capsules.

Precautions: Speak to a medical professional first with regards to your current healthcare plan. Side effects can include dizziness, diarrhea, vomiting, drowsiness, and dry mouth.

20. *Neurodegeneration*

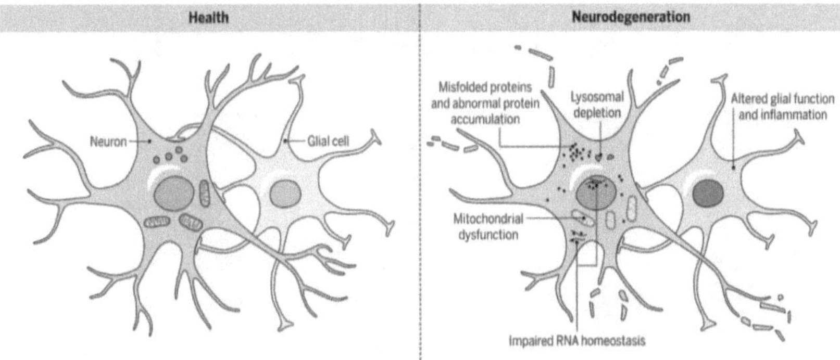

Neurodegeneration is the progressive loss of structure or function of neurons, including death of neurons. It's an age-associated degenerative illness that leads to loss of cognitive function and the human brain.

It is assumed that **symptoms include**:

- Being sick
- Feeling sick
- Difficulty with speech
- Ear bleeding
- Body numbness
- Limb paralysis
- Struggles with memory
- Difficulty concentrating
- High blood pressure
- Low heart rate
- Dilation of the pupils
- Irregular breathing

CBD is considered very promising for neurodegeneration by researchers (*pubmed.ncbi.nlm.nih.gov/19228180),* because of the calming effect it has on the nervous system. There are new studies being conducted all the time, so you can keep up to date with the latest information.

Dosage: You will need medical advice on this.

Application: You will need medical advice on this.

Precautions: You will need medical advice on this.

21. Huntington's Disease

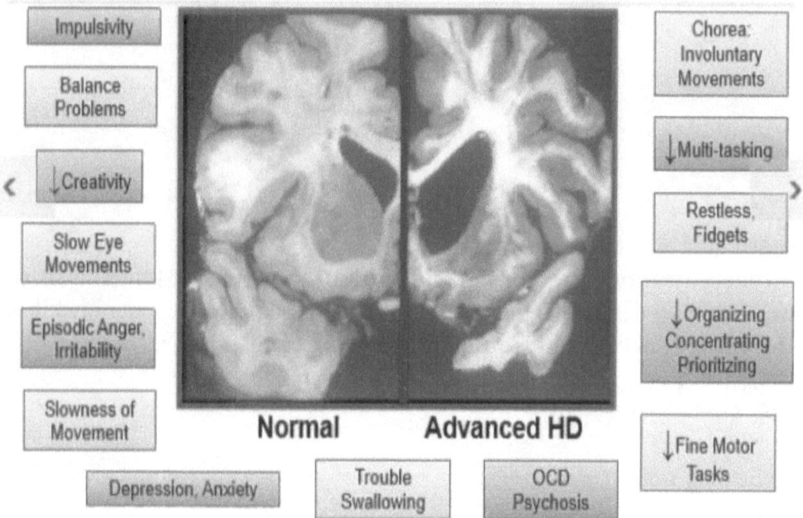

Huntington's disease is an inherited disorder that results in death of brain cells. The earliest symptoms are often subtle problems with mood or mental abilities. A general lack of coordination and an unsteady gait often follow.

If this is something you're worried about, **look out for:**

- Difficulty with swallowing or speech

- Impaired balance, posture, and gait

- Involuntary writing, jerking movement (also known as chorea)

- Muscle contracture (also known as dystonia) or other muscle problems, such as rigidity

- Slow, abnormal eye movements

CBD has been the subject of many studies that have found the CBD interacts with cannabinoid receptors in the body of the user; plus, the antioxidant properties help sufferers in a therapeutic way.

Dosage: Daily, over the course of six weeks, apply 10 mg of CBD oil per kg of body weight by mouth.

Application: Oil or capsules.

Precautions: Consult a medical professional with regards to your current healthcare plan. Side effects can include dizziness, fatigue, and dry mouth.

22. *Stroke*

A stroke is a serious life-threatening medical condition that occurs when the blood supply to part of the brain is cut off. This condition is an urgent medical emergency and immediate treatment must be sought out. The quicker action is taken, the less the damage will be.

The symptoms to look out for are:

- The face may have dropped to one side.

- It's difficult to lift both arms.

- Speech will be slurred.

CBD cannot stop a stroke from happening, but it can assist with the treatment in the crisis period immediately following. The neurodegenerative properties can trigger brain cell repair and generation. In use afterwards, it can also help a sufferer recover from the aftereffects.

Dosage: 0.25 mg to 0.5 mg of CBD oil per 1 pound of body weight once or twice per day for stroke recovery.

Application: Oil.

Precautions: Be aware of the side effects, particularly dizziness.

23. *Cancer*

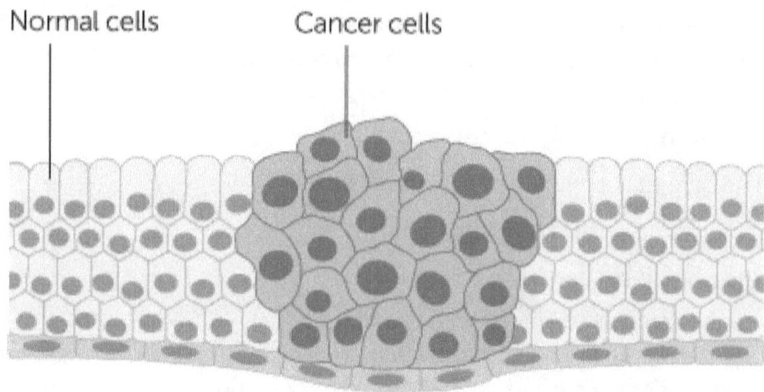

Cancer is a group of diseases involving abnormal cell growth with the potential to invade or spread to other parts of the body. These contrast with benign tumors, which do not spread to other parts of the body. Because it can affect any part of your body, it's difficult to know what to look out for, but upon seeing lumps, moles, bleeding, and any other symptoms that might appear very different, it's always best to go get checked out just to be on the safe side.

There has been a lot of research into the use of cannabidiol and the symptoms of cancer, and **it's been found that CBD can:**

- Cause a cell to die

- Stop cells from dividing

- Stop cells from developing new blood vessels

Dosage: You will need medical advice on this because dosage may vary from patient to patient. Most likely you will need a therapeutic dose which is between 50 mg and 800 mg of CBD per day.

Application: Oils or capsules.

Precautions: You will need to seek professional medical advice before applying CBD oil to ensure it works with your current medication. Side effects can include low blood pressure, dizziness, and fatigue.

24. Tumor

A tumor can be benign (not cancerous, no issues, doesn't need to be removed), premalignant (not yet cancerous, but might develop into that), or malignant (cancerous, which can spread or get worse). If this is something you suffer from, you might notice **the following symptoms**; in which case, you need to get medical intervention to see what the cause might be:

- Chills
- Fever and fever symptoms
- Loss of appetite
- Pain
- Sleep problem
- Weight loss

CBD has been found to actually reduce the size of a tumor (*cannabisclinicians.org/2011/07/24/cannabis-cancer-research*). Dr. Sean McAllister is the leading scientist in discovering that the ID-1 gene can be destroyed by CBD, which really helps to prevent tumors from growing.

Dosage: You will need to consult a medical professional first.

Application: Oil or capsules.

Precautions: Consult a medical professional before using. The side effects can be dizziness, hallucinations, and sickness.

25. *AIDS*

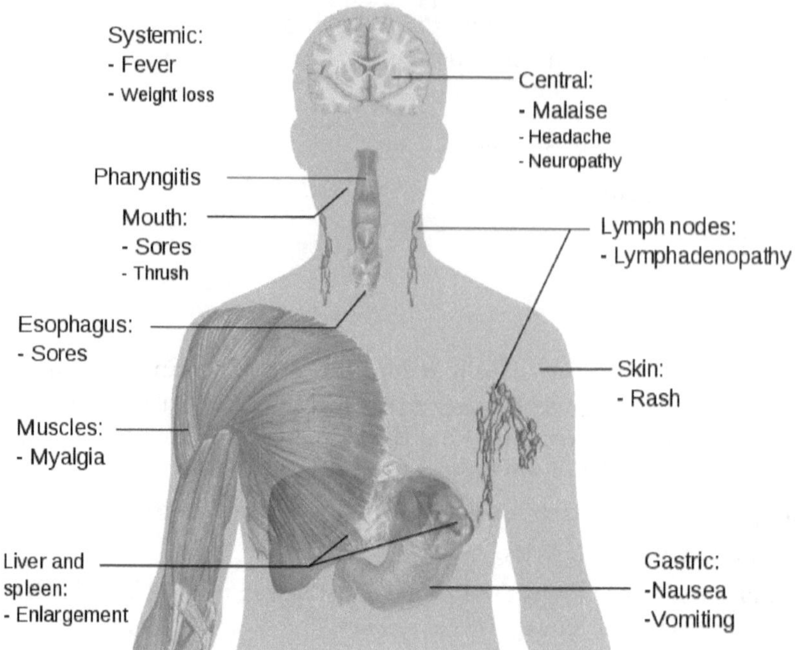

AIDS is a virus that attacks the immune system, which is our body's natural defense against illness. The virus destroys a type of white blood cell in the immune system called a T-helper cell and makes copies of itself inside these cells. T-helper cells are also referred to as CD4 cells. It's found in semen, blood, vaginal and anal fluids, and breast milk.

It's passed on through sweat, salvia, urine, sexual intercourse, injecting drugs, and pregnancy. **The symptoms of AIDS include:**

- Chronic fatigue

- Cough and shortness of breath

- Nausea

- Persistent diarrhea

- Rapid weight loss

- Recurring chills, fever, and night sweats

- Sores, lesions, or rashes in the nose or mouth, under the skin, or on the genitals

- Vomiting

CBD cannot cure AIDS, but it can help to relieve the symptoms of it. The pain, the loss of appetite, the difficulty sleeping, the inflammation – CBD can make everyday life easier to live.

Dosage: Start with 25 mg of CBD oil per day. Increase if needed. You might also want to look into other hemp products.

Application: Oil or capsules.

Precautions: Be aware of the side effects and consult a doctor first. These can be dry mouth, drowsiness, and light-headedness.

26. Anorexia

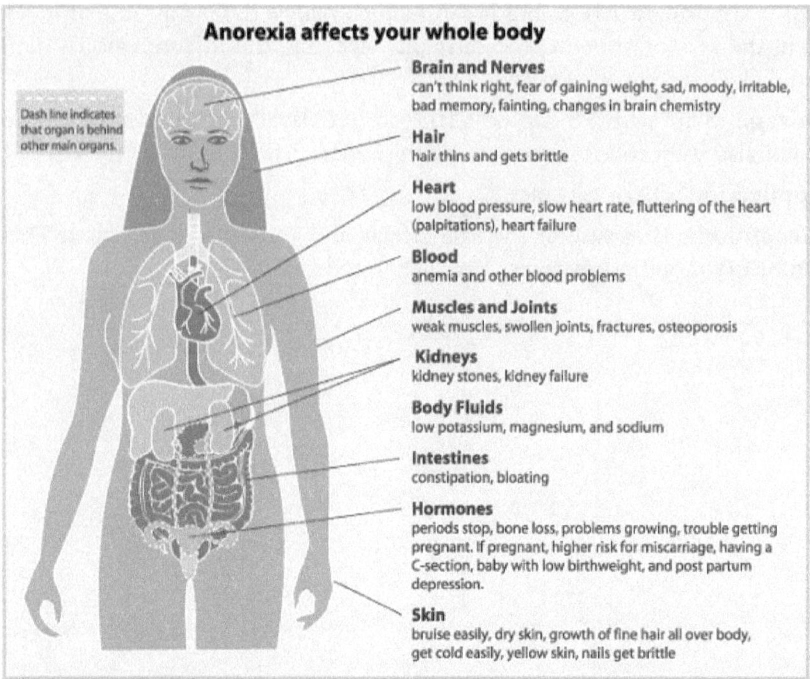

Anorexia is a serious mental illness where people are of low weight due to limiting their energy intake. Sufferers starve their bodies because they have distorted images of their bodies. **The symptoms to look out for** are as follows:

- Teenagers, under 18, whose height and weight are too low for their age

- Adults with a body mass index (BMI) that is too low

- Skipping meals, eating too little, or choosing not to eat any foods seen as 'fattening'

- Seeing yourself as fat even when you are at a healthy weight or may be underweight

- Using appetite suppressants to inhibit your hunger urges

- Menstrual periods stop for women too young to have reached menopause or starting too late for younger girls and young adults

- Displaying physical problems, such as dry skin, hair loss, dizziness, or light-headedness

It's a very serious condition that needs medical intervention sooner rather than later, before it gets worse. Sufferers can end up hospitalized, and the disease can even become fatal. Anorexia is linked to endocannabinoid deficiency, so using CBD can help improve the nervous system, the appetite, and balance the psychoactive effects. It won't cure the underlying issues, but it can help.

TIP: Consistency works best. Be patient. If you stick with the dose that improves your condition, in 2 -3 months it will be better yet.

Dosage: 25-1,000 mg per day dependent on weight.

Application: Oil or vape.

Precautions: Be aware of the side effects, in particular dizziness and diarrhea, and consult a medical professional first. Particularly if taking other medication.

27. *Osteoporosis*

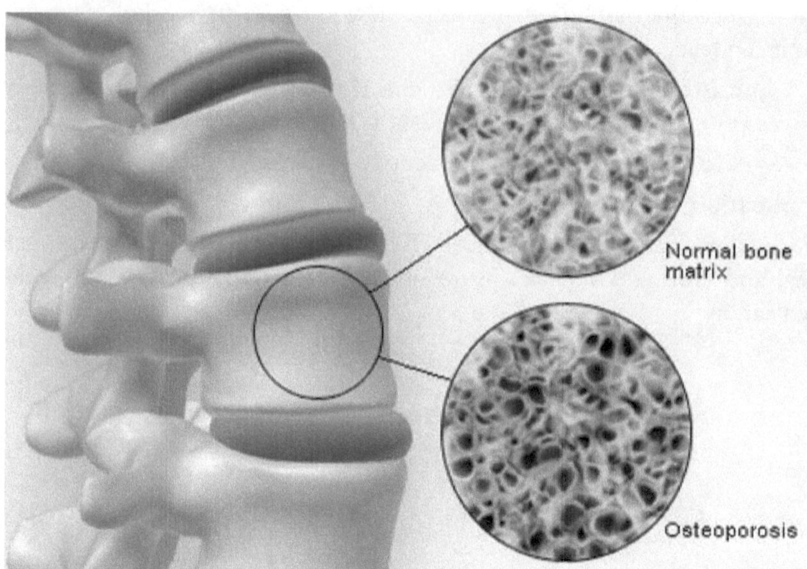

Osteoporosis is a condition that weakens bones, making them fragile and more likely to break. It develops slowly over several years and is often only diagnosed when a minor fall or sudden impact causes a bone fracture. The causes of this can be long-term use of certain medications, a family history, drinking, and smoking. You will need to request a DEXA scan if this is something you suspect you might have.

It is suggested for you to **look out for**:

- Unexplained back pain that may be caused by a collapsed or fractured vertebra

- Experiencing a loss in height over time

- Posture appears stooped

- Bone fractures that occur too easily

A study (at *ncbi.nlm.nih.gov/pmc/articles/PMC3423262*) has discovered that:

- Cannabinoid receptors, CB1, CB2, and orphan receptor GPR55, exist within the bone cells. Studies have shown that these receptors and endocannabinoids have an impact on osteoporosis development.

- By blocking the aforementioned receptors, researchers were able to suppress the resorption of bones in adult mice. This resulted in an increase of bone mass and protected the mice against additional bone loss. As such, they have suggested the use of CBD, which is an inverse antagonist to the receptors, to help combat osteoporosis.

- From another study, an increase in spongy (or trabecular) bone and outer surface (or cortical) was discovered after blocking GPR55's effect. The mice experienced better protection against age-related bone loss and put on weight after their GPR55 receptors were knocked out. Based on that, scientists have concluded there are benefits for osteoporosis patients by administering CBD.

Dosage: 10 mg to 100 mg per day. (*hemppedia.org/cbd-for-osteoporosis*)

Application: Oil or capsules.

Precautions: Consult a medical professional first with regards to your current healthcare plan. You will want to be aware of side effects such as dizziness, weakness, and fatigue.

28. *Dyskinesia*

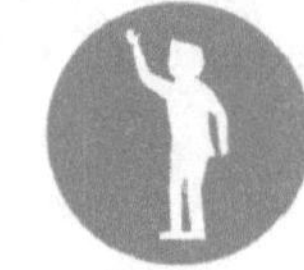

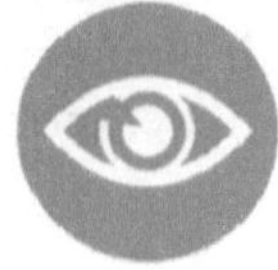

Know the Signs of TD

Symptoms May Range from Mild to Severe

Movements of the Mouth
Such as frowning, sticking out tongue, lip smacking, puckering, and pursing

Rapid Movements of the Body
Commonly in the arms, legs, and trunk

Face
Disfigured facial features such as drooping of the mouth or eyes

Eyes
Rapid blinking

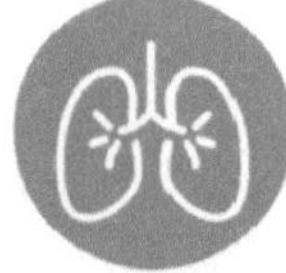
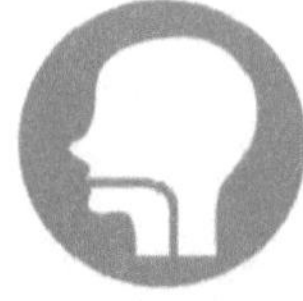

Difficulty Breathing

Difficulty Swallowing

Difficulty Speaking

MHA B4Stage4 SOURCES
Keshavan, M. S. (1992). Drug-induced dysfunction in psychia try. New York: Hemisphere publ. Corporation.

Dyskinesia is an abnormal, uncontrolled, involuntary movement. It can affect one body part, such as an arm, leg or the head, or it can spread over the entire body. Dyskinesia can look like fidgeting, writhing, wriggling, head bobbing or body swaying.

As it's an attack on the nervous system, CBD can be very useful when managing the symptoms of it, as many studies show. It's shown to calm down the involuntary movements of the body.

Dosage: Start with 25 mg of CBD oil per day, increase if needed. Other hemp products, such as seeds, can be beneficial.

Application: Oil or capsules.

Precautions: Do not take without consulting a medical professional first. The oil can slow the effects of your current medication. You may also experience drowsiness and diarrhea.

29. *Diabetes*

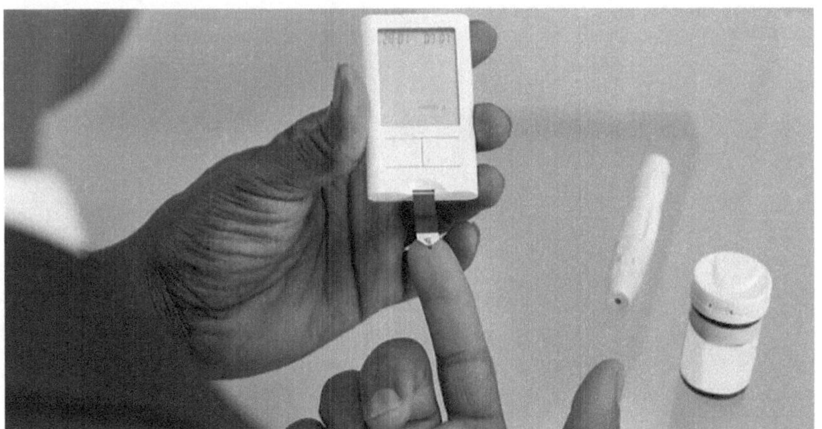

Diabetes is a group of metabolic disorders in which there are high blood sugar levels over a prolonged period. Symptoms of high blood sugar include frequent urination, increased thirst, and increased hunger. If left untreated, diabetes can cause many complications.

Diabetes comes in **two types:**

- *Type 1 diabetes* – the immune system attacks, then destroys, the cells producing insulin

- *Type 2 diabetes* – the body isn't producing enough insulin, or if the body does produce enough insulin, the cells don't react to it

Symptoms to look out for include:

- Blurred vision

- Feeling very thirsty

- Feeling very tired

- Itching around vagina or penis, frequent bouts of thrush

- Urinating more frequently, especially at night

- Weight or muscle bulk loss

- Wounds or cuts heal more slowly

Studies have shown that the work that CBD does in the pancreas is extremely beneficial to diabetes sufferers. It's also useful for inflammation, sugar buildup, and metabolism. Nerve damage can also be found in diabetes sufferers. CBD can reduce this damage up to 30%.

Dosage: 100 mg of CBD oil twice daily for type 2 diabetes or 100-200 mg per day vaping.

Application: Oil, capsules, or vape.

Precautions: Be aware of the side effects. These can include digestive issues, drowsiness, and restlessness.

30. *Kidney Disease*

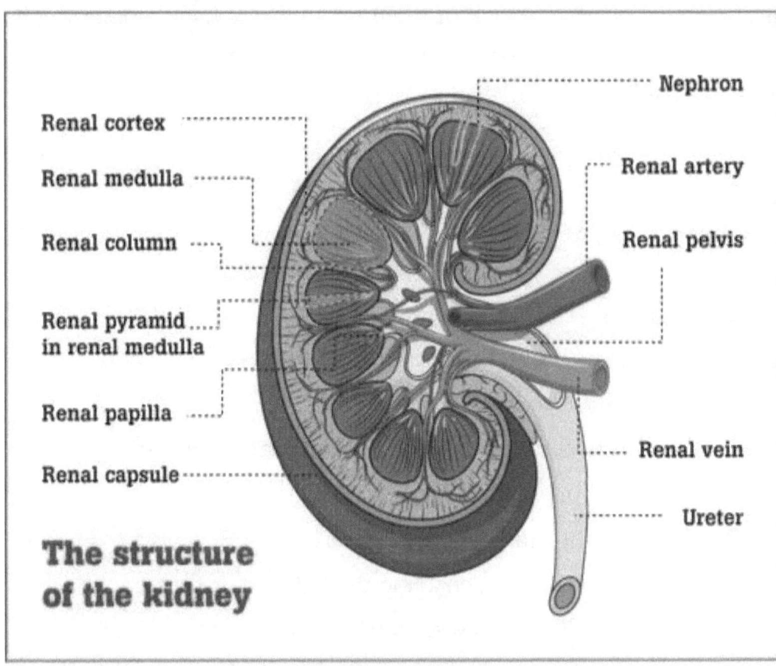

**The structure
of the kidney**

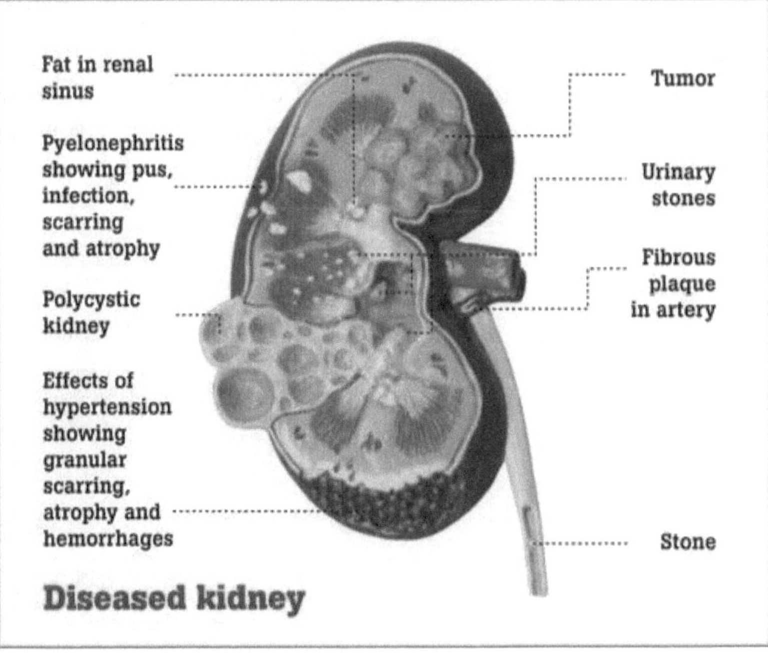

Diseased kidney

Kidney disease is a long-term condition where the kidneys don't work as they should. This condition can escalate and eventually the kidneys may stop working altogether. A few of the causes include high cholesterol, long-term use of specific medications, high blood pressure, and many more.

Symptoms include:

- Fatigue

- Swollen ankles and feet

- Struggling with breathing

- Sickness

- Blood in urine

Preliminary tests into CBD use in kidney disease have seen:

- Improved kidney function

- Maintained safe cholesterol levels, keeping the heart safe

- Lowered blood pressure

- Alleviated pressure and enhanced sleep

- Boosted immune system, enabling the fight against infections

- Repaired damaged organs with anti-inflammatory properties

Dosage: 20-40 mg of CDB oil three times daily. Other hemp products may as well be beneficial.

Application: Oil or capsules.

Precautions: Consult a medical professional with regards to your current healthcare plan. This can slow down the effects of your medication. It can also cause dry mouth, low blood pressure, and drowsiness.

31. *Liver Disease*

Liver, Gallbladder, Pancreas and Bile Passage

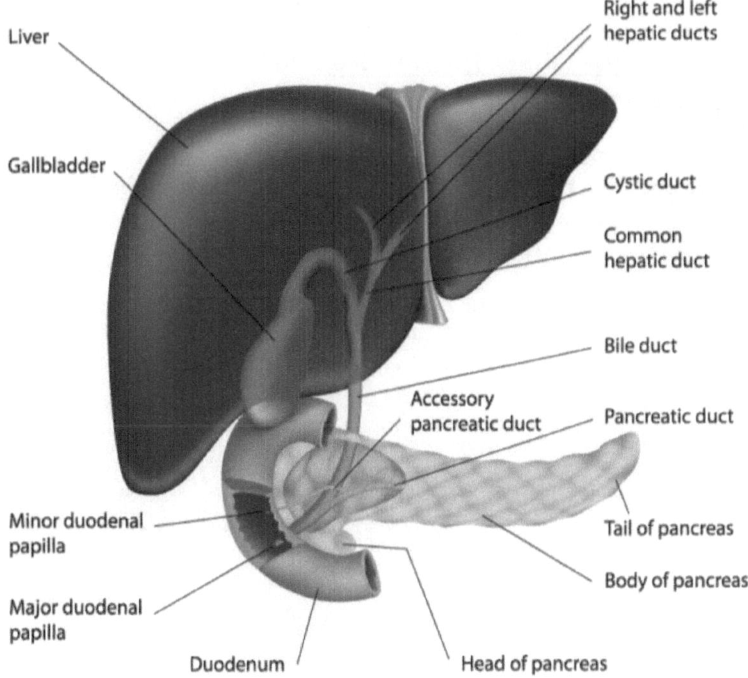

These are **different diseases that affect the liver:**

- Primary biliary cirrhosis – could be caused by an immune system problem

- Haemochromatosis – an inherited gene that runs in families, being passed from parent to child

- Hepatitis – can be caused by the regular, excessive drinking of alcohol or catching a viral infection

- Non-alcoholic fatty liver disease – being obese (very overweight) can cause fat buildup in the liver

- Alcohol-related liver disease – caused by regular, excessive drinking of alcohol

Experiencing the symptoms means the damage has already been done, and you must seek medical assistance immediately. They include:

- Chronic fatigue, weakness

- Jaundice (whites of the eyes and skin appear yellow)
- Reduced libido (sex drive)
- Weight loss, caused by loss of appetite

CBD has been proven to improve the quality of life for people with liver disease. The oil works with the endocannabinoid system in the body to reduce inflammation, dull the pain, and manage cell damage (*ncbi.nlm.nih.gov/pmc/articles/PMC3057300*)

Dosage: 600-1,200 mg of CBD oil per day.

Application: Oil or capsules.

Precautions: Don't take until you've consulted with a medical professional first. It can slow down the absorption of your other medication. You might also experience weakness, fatigue, and diarrhea.

32. Heart Health

The 4 Numbers
You Need To Know For
Heart Health

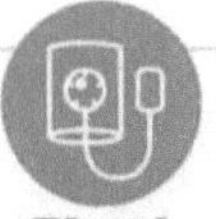

Blood Pressure

WHAT IT IS The force of your blood pressing against artery walls

IDEAL GOAL Less than 120/80 mm Hg

WHY High blood pressure, defined as 140/90 mm Hg and above, increases your risk of strokes and heart attacks.

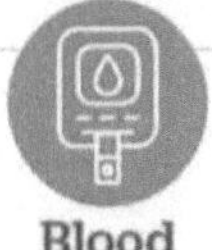

Blood Sugar

WHAT IT IS The amount of sugar (or glucose) in your blood, measured by hemoglobin A1c and/or fasting blood glucose tests

IDEAL GOAL HbA1c less than 5.7%; fasting glucose less than 126 mg/dL

WHY Diabetes is diagnosed when HbA1c is 6.5% or higher and/or fasting glucose is 126 mg/dL or higher. Too-high sugar levels can damage blood vessels, making you more susceptible to heart disease.

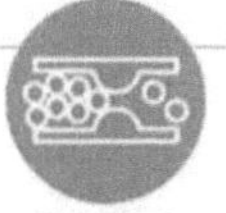

Blood Cholesterol

WHAT IT IS A fat-like, waxy substance in the blood

IDEAL GOAL *Total cholesterol:* Less than 200 mg/dL, *Triglycerides:* Less than 150 mg/dL, *"Good" HDL cholesterol:* Greater than 60 mg/dL, *"Bad" LDL cholesterol:* Less than 100 mg/dL

WHY Higher levels of cholesterol may block blood flow to the heart.

Body Mass Index

WHAT IT IS A measure of body fat calculated using your height and weight

IDEAL GOAL 18.5 to 24.9

WHY Excess bodyweight (a BMI of 25 and above is considered overweight; 30 and above is considered obese) increases heart disease risk, especially when waist circumference goes up.

When something is wrong with your heart health, it might be angina, a heart attack, or heart failure. It can be caused by diabetes, high cholesterol, and high blood pressure. You can help to prevent this by exercising regularly, stopping smoking, or taking medication.

Studies have shown that CBD helps relax the arterial walls, which prevents inflammation and makes the blood flow easier, slowing down any damage.

Dosage: 20-300 mg of CBD oil per day, depending on weight.

Application: Oil or capsules.

Precautions: Always consult a medical professional first. Side effects may include hypotension, dry mouth, light-headedness, dizziness, and tiredness.

33. Hepatitis C

Effects of Hepatitis C[1,2]

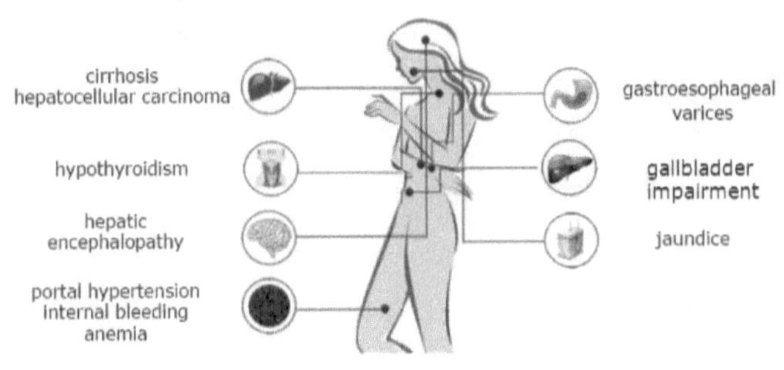

Hepatitis C is a virus that can infect the liver. If left untreated, it can sometimes cause serious and potentially life-threatening damage to the liver over many years. It's transferred by the blood of an infectious person through drug use, razors, and unprotected sex. **The symptoms include:**

- Abdominal pain

- Chronic fatigue

- Feeling and being sick

- Fever and flu-like symptoms, for instance, muscle aches

- Loss of appetite

CBD has been studied a lot (*ncbi.nlm.nih.gov/pmc/articles/PMC5330095*) to see how it works with hepatitis C, and the results have displayed very positive effects against the virus attacking the liver cells and the inflammation that follows.

Dosage: Start with 50-60 mg of CBD oil per day for symptomatic relief, and increase if needed (*cbdnhemp.com/cbd/benefits/cbd-oil-benefit-hepatitis-c*). Other hemp products can be also beneficial.

Application: Oil, capsules, and vape.

Precautions: Be aware of the side effects. These can include slow absorption of your current medication, drowsiness, and digestive issues.

34. Tapering Off Opioids

Tapering off opioids gets much harder the longer you are taking the drugs. These powerful painkillers are touted as the most effective medicinal treatment against acute, short-term pain, but if the pain you're suffering takes longer to heal, the opioids will stop being as effective, meaning you'll need to increase your dosage, only strengthening your body's addiction to it.

The withdrawal symptoms include:

- Anxiety or restlessness
- Blood pressure fluctuations
- Confusion
- Diarrhea, nausea, or vomiting
- Drowsiness
- Fevers or sweating
- Increased pain
- Rapid heart rate
- Seizures or hallucinations – hearing, seeing, or feeling things that aren't real
- Tremors
- Trouble sleeping

These side effects are unpleasant, which is where CBD can come into play. Not only is it a great replacement for the pain-killer effect that the opioids have, it'll calm down the nasty withdrawal effects, making it a much easier transition for you.

There are many online stories for you to read from real patients making this transition.

Dosage: This will depend on the dosage of your opioids. Consult a medical professional about this first. They will often recommend you start with 25 mg of CBD oil per day.

Application: Oil, capsules, or vape.

Precautions: Be aware of the side effects, which may include dry mouth, drowsiness, digestive issues, and restlessness.

35. Substance Abuse

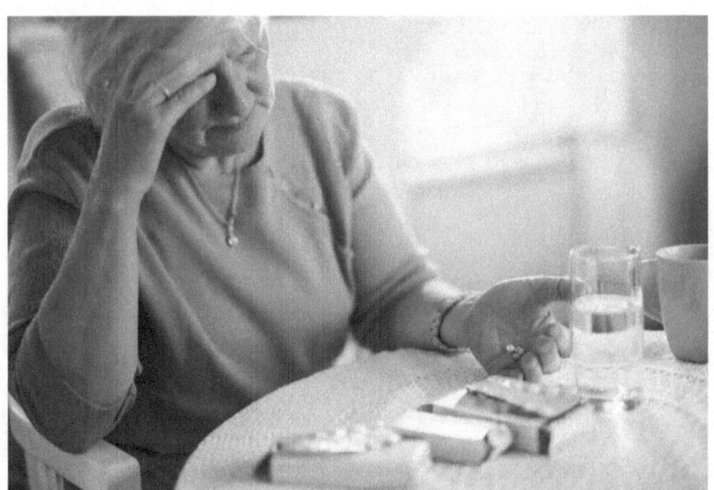

Substance abuse is taking something illegal or using a substance in the wrong way. The addiction is a disease that affects each individual sufferer in a different way. Misuse of alcohol, drugs, prescription medication, and many more substances can cause this issue.

It is suggested that **the signs to look out for include**:

- Change your friends frequently
- Eat more or less than usual
- Experience problems with family or at work
- Lack of interest in things you once loved
- Sleep at unusual hours
- Spend more time alone than normal
- Stop practicing self-care
- Switch rapidly between feeling bad and good

Many researchers have looked into the effect CBD can have on people who are in recovery, and it's been found to reduce the number of relapses. It also reduces anxiety, pain, inflammation and can even help to repair the damage done to a sufferer's brain.

Dosage: This will depend on the substance. Consult a medical professional about this first, as they will be able to give you an accurate individual evaluation.

Application: Oil, capsules, or vape.

Precautions: Be aware of the side effects, which may include tiredness, diarrhea, and weakness.

36. *Quitting Smoking*

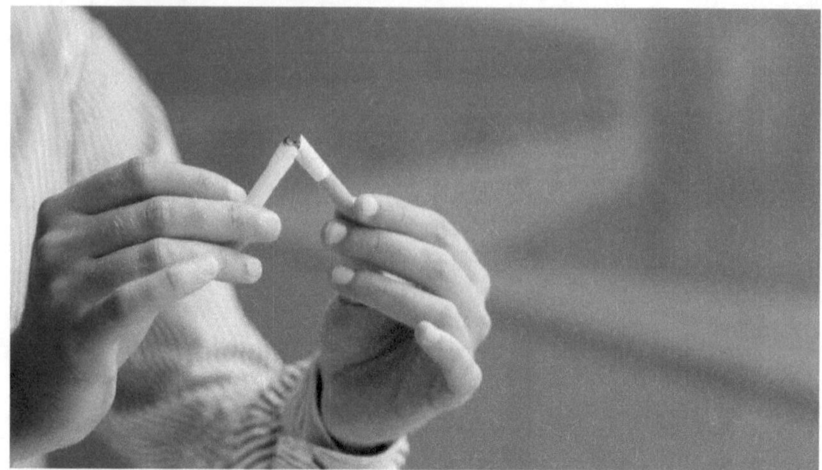

Quitting smoking is a huge challenge for those who are addicted to it. It is assumed **this is because**:

- Cigarettes contain nicotine, and it's difficult to overcome a physical addiction to it. Nicotine is a natural substance in tobacco and is highly addictive. It may be due to how quickly it can travel to the brain after it is inhaled. This often causes a feeling of temporary stress relief and/or relaxation. Also, nicotine can elevate your heart rate and mood. However, these feelings are only temporary. Once your body processes the drug, you begin to have cravings for another cigarette.

- This new craving can begin as soon as you finish smoking a cigarette. Your body can immediately start to show signs of withdrawal from the nicotine. Wanting to overcome these symptoms, the craving for another cigarette begins, which starts the never-ending cycle of dependency.

- Finding new avenues for handling stress can be challenging. Especially if you are reaching for a cigarette as soon as you feel anxious or stressed. No matter where the stress comes from, your relationships, responsibilities, emotional burdens, or the fast pace of daily living, it can make you look for the fastest and easiest source of relief.

But it's an essential challenge to overcome because it'll make your lungs breathe easier, it'll give you more energy, and you'll live much longer. Everyone knows the benefits of quitting smoking, but sometimes it isn't the easiest thing to do. This is where CBD can come into play.

The cannabidiol can replace the nicotine, as shown by a study conducted by the University of London (*news.herbapproach.com/done-smoker-quit-cigarettes-cbd*). Users also felt a reduction in stress, anxiety, as well as having that oral fixation removed.

Most of the clinical trials have shown that CBD can reduce nicotine addiction and have actually reduced the number of cigarettes smoked by 40 percent.

Dosage: Start with 0.5 ml of CBD oil taken twice daily 12 hours apart and continue for 3 weeks (*cannabisace.com/what-is-cbd/cbd-oil-quit-smoking-cigarettes*).

Application: Oil.

Precautions: Be aware of the side effects, which can include fatigue, dizziness, and drowsiness.

37. Anxiety

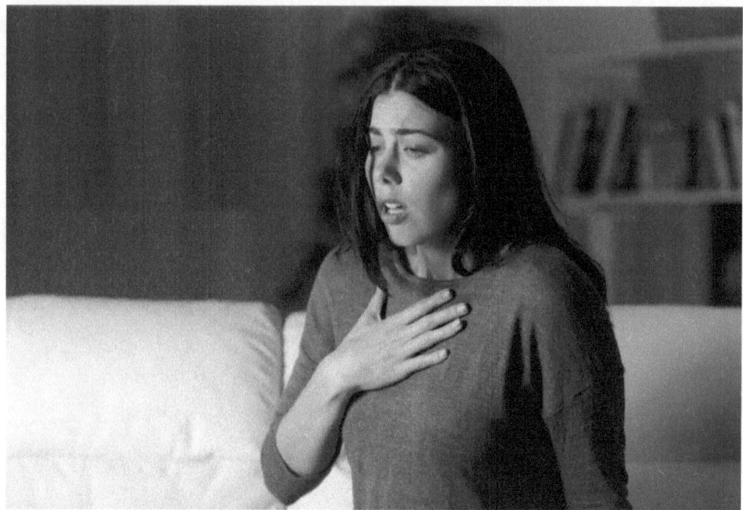

Anxiety is a feeling of unease, such as worry or fear, that can be mild or severe. While this is something that everyone experiences from time to time when stressful situations arise, anxiety sufferers find it much harder to control even the smallest of worries. This can manifest itself as post-traumatic stress disorder, various phobias, panic disorder, or social anxiety disorder, among others.

Did you know that anxiety disorders today affect 18.1 percent of adults in the US?

Anxiety is caused by:

- Genes inherited from parents can make you five times more likely to develop general anxiety disorder

- History of substance, drug or alcohol, abuse/misuse

- History of traumatic or stressful life experiences, such as bullying or abuse

- Imbalance in brain chemistry, specifically serotonin or noradrenaline that play a role in regulating mood

- Painful, long-term health conditions, such as nerve damage or arthritis

- Overactivity in regions of the brain regulating behavior and emotions

CBD and anxiety have been studied a lot together (*leafly.com/news/health/cbd-for-treating-anxiety*), and it's been discovered that the oil works well with the 5-HT1A to help boost serotonin (the happiness hormone). It can also calm the nervous system, lower blood pressure, and decrease discomfort.

Did you know that 20 percent of Americans that use CBD products, use it for anxiety symptoms?

TIP: CBD has been found to significantly reduce cognitive impairment and discomfort in speech performance, so if you intend to speak in public, CBD oil can significantly decrease angst surrounding it.

Dosage: 300-600 mg of CDB oil. For best results, take CBD oil first thing in the morning, and repeat around lunch time.

Application: Oil, capsules, or vape.

Precautions: Be aware of the side effects, which can include gastrointestinal discomfort, sleeplessness, dry mouth, and dizziness.

38. Depression

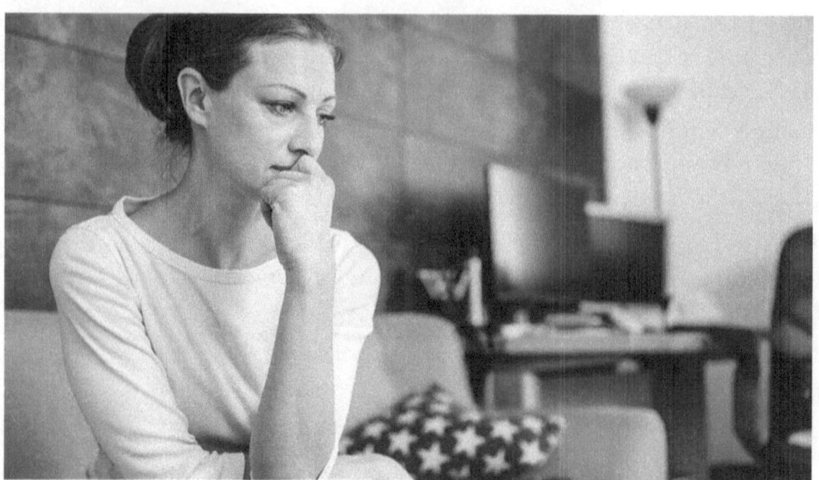

Depression is more than simply feeling unhappy or fed up for a few days. Most people go through periods of feeling down, but when you're depressed you feel persistently sad for weeks or months, rather than just a few days. This can be mild (minor impact on daily life), moderate (impact on every day), or severe (makes it impossible to get through everyday life).

Symptoms are different from person to person, and affect you psychologically, physically, and socially, as shown by this **list of possible symptoms**:

- Avoiding contact with friends and other social activity
- Anxious or worried feelings
- Constant sadness or low mood
- Constipation
- Difficulty making decisions
- Difficulty with family and work life
- Difficulty with sleeping, and then waking up
- Feeling guilt-ridden
- Feeling helpless and hopeless
- Feeling intolerant of others and irritable
- Feeling tearful
- Fluctuations in appetite and weight
- Fluctuations in menstrual cycle
- Having low self-esteem

- Having no motivation or interest
- Having thoughts of suicide or self-harm
- Lack of energy
- Low or loss of libido (sex drive)
- Neglecting hobbies and interests
- Not feeling any enjoyment from life
- Speaking or moving more slowly
- Unexplained pains and body aches

While CBD cannot cure depression, you will need to seek medical intervention for that, it can assist with the symptoms, making day to day living a little bit more bearable. Disturbed sleep, anxiety, low moods, and lack of energy can be improved using CBD.

Dosage: 40-600 mg per day, depending on your weight and needs.

Application: Oil, capsules, vape, or topical application.

Precautions: Consult a medical professional first with regards to your current healthcare plan. It can slow the effects of any current medication you're on. You may also experience dizzy spells, fatigue, and digestive issues.

39. *Bipolar*

BIPOLAR DISORDER FACTS

1 2% OF THE UK POPULATION

In a screening for the NHS, 2% of the UK screened positive to suffering with Bipolar Disorder, with similar rates found between male and female patients.

2 6TH LEADING DISABILITY

Bipolar Disorder is the 6th leading mental health disability.

3 60% WITHOUT TREATMENT

Of all those screened by the NHS, 60% of positive Bipolar Disorder sufferers were currently without any form of treatment, either medical or psychological.

4 COMMON IN YOUNG PEOPLE

3.4% of those between 16-24 screened positive for bipolar disorder, which is over 8 times more than those between 65-74 who only had a rate of 0.4%.

5 1-5% WORLDWIDE AVERAGE

Average worldwide prevalence can be anywhere from 1% to 5% of the overall population.

Bipolar disorder, previously known as manic depression, is a mental disorder that causes periods of depression and periods of abnormally elevated mood. The elevated mood is significant and is known as mania or hypomania, depending on its severity, or whether symptoms of psychosis are present.

The constant highs and lows that come with this disorder can be very hard to live with. The NHS reports **the following tips can help:**

- Take medication to assist with the manic and depression periods

- Seek out psychological therapy, such as talk therapy, which can help you cope with depression by providing guidance on how to improve coping mechanisms and relationships

- Work toward awareness for signs of and what triggers the depression and mania episodes

- Follow lifestyle advice by performing regular exercise, pursuing activities you enjoy to generate a sense of achievement, getting more sleep, and improving your diet

CBD can help to improve cognitive functions and alleviate periods of depression and mania. In fact, some studies have found that people with bipolar using CBD felt less pain, less anxiety, and positive effects to their neuroprotective system.

Dosage: Start with 125 mg of CBD oil per day and increase if needed.

Application: Oil or capsules.

Precautions: Be aware of the side effects, which can include dry mouth, fatigue, and diarrhea.

40. *Insomnia*

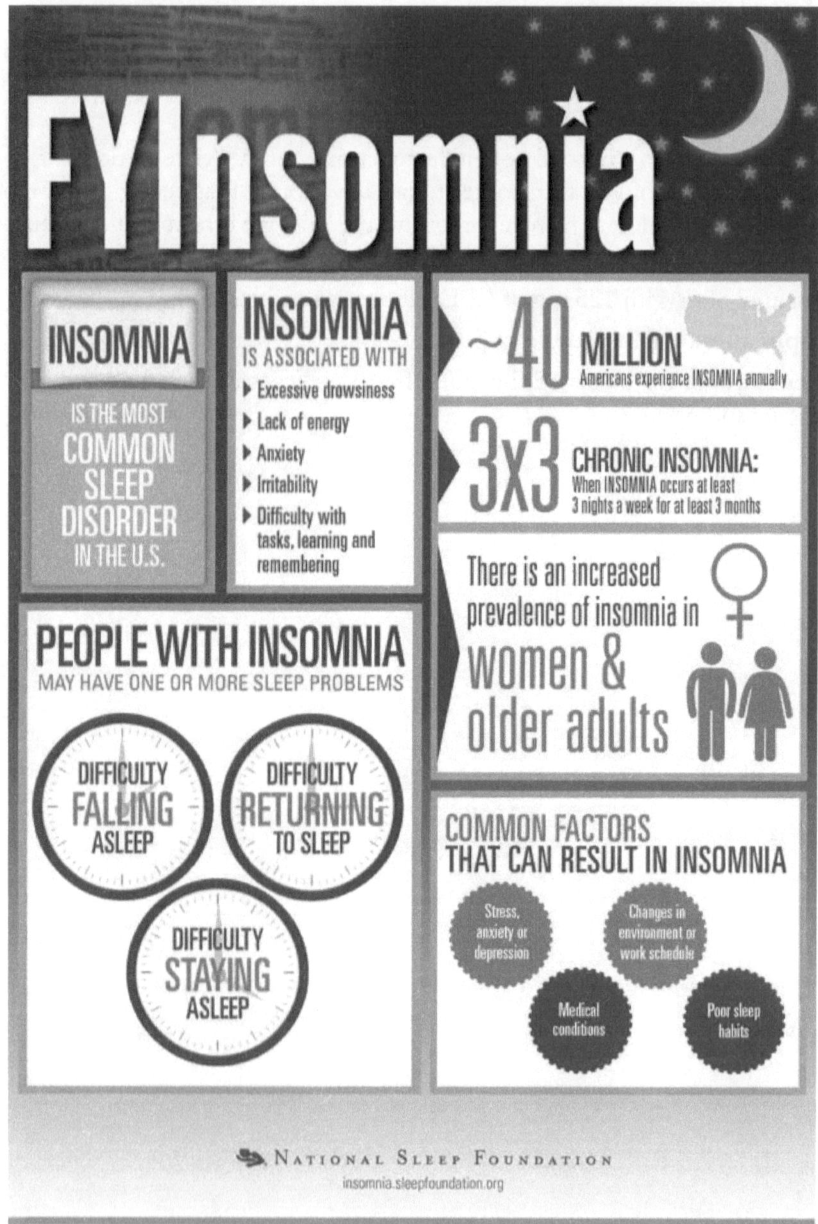

Insomnia is a sleep disorder where people have trouble sleeping. They may have difficulty falling asleep or staying asleep as long as desired. You need 7 to 9 hours per night, so if that isn't happening, you might have insomnia.

Other signs include:

- Difficulty concentrating during the day due to fatigue
- Difficulty falling asleep
- Feel tired and irritable during the day
- Find it hard to nap during the day even though you're tired
- Lie awake at night
- Still feel tired after waking up
- Wake up early and can't fall back to sleep
- Wake up several times during the night

It can be caused by many things but **the most common reasons are**:

- Alcohol, nicotine, or caffeine
- Anxiety, stress, or depression
- Jet lag
- Recreational drugs, such as ecstasy or cocaine
- Room temperature is too hot or cold
- Shift work
- Too noisy
- Uncomfortable beds

You can help yourself by getting into a sleep routine; avoiding caffeine, alcohol, and cigarettes after 6:00 p.m.; relaxing, exercising more, and making sure that you're comfortable. CBD oil also helps to promote better sleep because of the calming properties scientists have discovered. The change in the activity of neurotransmitters, hormones, and other cells throughout the brain and body are all very positive for getting a better night of sleep.

Dosage: 40-160 mg of CBD oil by mouth daily.

TIP: Some CBD dosing experiments have shown that small doses of CBD (less than 10 mg) have an "active" effect, which means it actually helps you stay active and focused, while large doses (more than 20 mg) have the opposite – sedation effect. Aim for the heavy dose of CBD oil, if the goal is to improve your sleep.

Application: Oil or capsules.

Precautions: Be aware of the side effects, which can include restlessness and fatigue.

41. PTSD

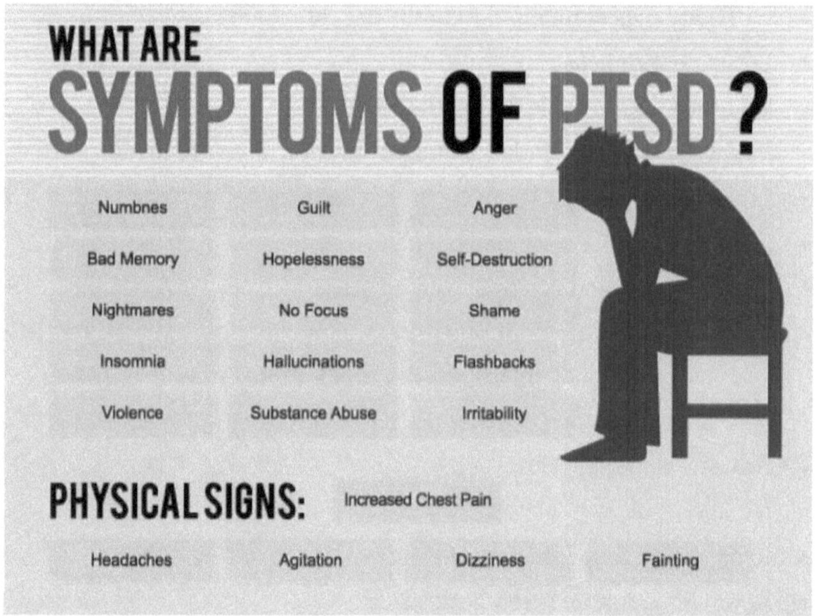

Post-traumatic stress disorder is an anxiety disorder caused by very stressful, frightening or distressing events. Examples of 'frightening or distressing events' are natural disasters, violence, military active duty or combat, physical assault, or many more. It may not come about right away after the incident, and it affects everyone in very different ways.

The treatment of this disorder is often done through therapy, medication, and a lot of waiting, which can leave sufferers very frustrated and wanting to help themselves. Luckily, there has been a lot of testing into the use of CBD to help PTSD (*projectcbd.org/hub/ptsd*). While it cannot get rid of the problem, it can help with the side effects. Using CBD can calm the CB1 and CB2 receptors in the body's central nervous system, alleviating depression, stress, and sleep problems.

Dosage: Start with 350 mg of CBD oil per day. Consult a medical professional if you need a larger dose.

Application: Oils, capsules, or vape.

Precautions: Consult with a medical professional beforehand with regards to your current healthcare plan. It can slow the effects of your current medication. You may also experience dizziness, dry mouth, and digestive troubles.

42. *ADHD*

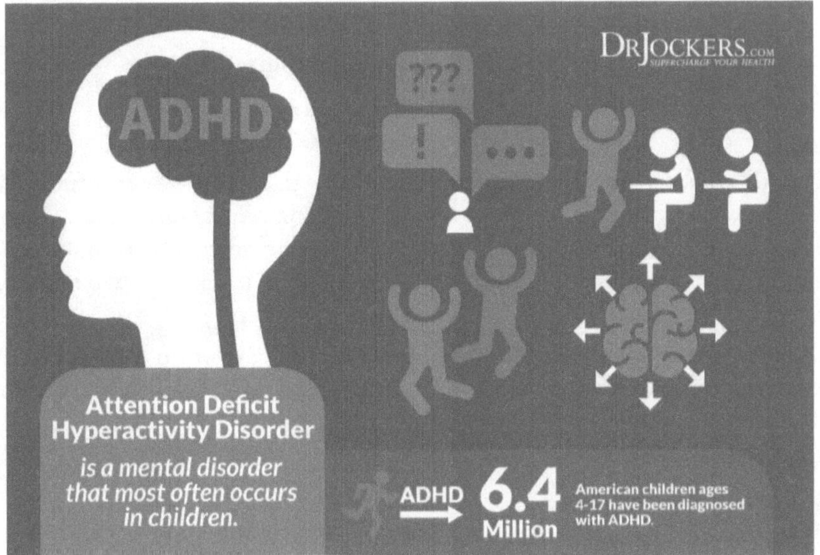

Attention deficit hyperactivity disorder (ADHD) is a group of behavioral symptoms that include inattentiveness, hyperactivity and impulsiveness. Symptoms of ADHD tend to be noticed at an early age and may become more noticeable when a child's circumstances change, such as when they start school.

While children often go through restlessness or inattentive phases, **these traits are much worse in sufferers of ADHD**:

- Acting without thinking or making careless mistakes
- Appearing unable to carry out instructions or to listen
- Appearing forgetful or misplacing things
- Constantly changing tasks or activities
- Constantly fidgeting
- Distracted easily or has a short attention span
- Excessive physical movement
- Excessive talking
- Has difficulty organizing tasks
- Impulsiveness and hyperactivity
- Unable to sit still in quiet or calm environment
- Unable to concentrate on activities or tasks

- Unable to follow through with time-consuming or tedious tasks

- Unable to practice patience or calmly wait for their turn

- Unable to hold conversations without interrupting

- Very reckless, acting with little to no sense of danger

While CBD cannot cure this issue, it can help improve a sufferer's quality of life. ADHD is a neurodevelopmental disorder that can make it difficult to control what you focus on, and it's also often combined with anxiety. Many users have found that the results were instantaneous and noticeable (*adhdboss.com/cbd-oil-adhd*). Other studies have found it can also help with the negative symptoms of the illness, such as lack of sleep.

Dosage: Between 40 and 100 mg of CBD oil per day for up to 3 weeks. 20 to 25 mg per day is enough for maintenance dosing to keep the symptoms at bay.

Application: Oil, or they can be found in a gummy form (e.g. *id-weeds.com/best-cbd-gummies*).

Precautions: Get advice from a medical professional for any age child, particularly one under 12 years old. Side effects can include fatigue, restlessness, and digestive problems.

43. Acne

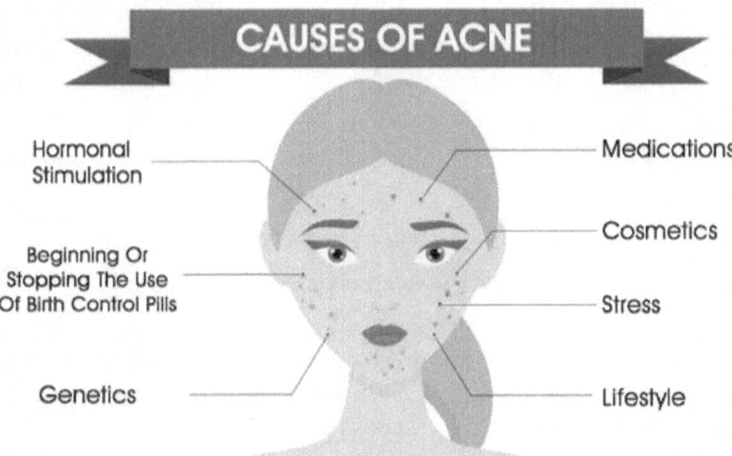

Acne is a long-term skin disease that occurs when hair follicles are clogged with dead skin cells and oil from the skin. It is characterized by blackheads or whiteheads, pimples, oily skin, and possible scarring. It can develop on your chest, back, and face.

The spots can be characterized by:

- Blackheads – small bumps, black or yellow in color, develop on the skin; they appear black due to the hair follicle lining producing that color

- Cysts – these large lumps are the most severe spot caused by acne; they are pus-filled, have a similar appearance to boils, and have greatest risk of leaving permanent scars

- Nodules – hard, large lumps, that can be painful, appear beneath the skin's surface

- Papules – tiny bumps in a red color that can feel sore or tender

- Pustules – looks similar to papules, except for the white point in the center that is generated by a buildup of pus

- Whiteheads – looks similar to the blackhead, but feels firmer and may not empty with applied pressure

To help with this condition, you can:

- Avoid using too much cosmetic or makeup products. Look for water-based makeup that is labeled 'non-comedogenic,' meaning it is less likely to block pores.

- Wash the breakout area using a mild cleanser or soap with lukewarm water. Extremely cold or hot water can make symptoms worse.

- But, don't wash the affected areas more than twice per day. Washing too often will further irritate the skin and can make symptoms worse.

- Avoid squeezing blackheads or 'popping' acne breakouts. This can cause permanent scarring, additional breakouts, and make symptoms worse.

- Wash off all of your makeup before going to sleep.

- Regularly wash your hair and keep it pinned back and away from your face.

- Exercising doesn't have an effect on acne, but it does improve self-esteem and mood. However, sweat can irritate and generate acne, so shower as soon as you finish exercising.

- If you have dry skin, apply a water-based, fragrance-free emollient.

CBD also has proven positive effects when it comes to acne. The cannabinoids slow down the production of sebum, which leads to less oily skin, resulting in less acne. Many users have also confirmed that it left their skin much clearer (e.g. *hemptouch.com/blog/interview-cbd-oil-cleared-my-skin-of-acne*).

TIP: Look for CBD skin care in stable packaging - no jars, clear bottles or any component that exposes this delicate plant ingredient to a lot of light or air, which cause it to become less effective.

Dosage: This will depend on your skin condition. Consult a medical professional first as they will be able to give you the correct advice according to your individual needs.

Application: Oil, capsules, or topically applied to the affected area.

Precautions: Be aware of the side effects, which can include dizziness, tiredness, and stomach troubles.

44. Psoriasis

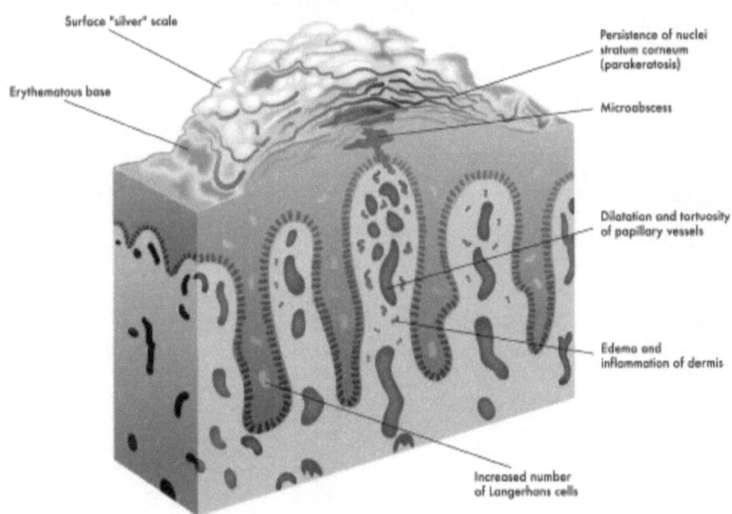

Psoriasis is a skin condition that causes red, flaky, crusty patches of skin covered with silvery scales. These patches normally appear on your elbows, knees, scalp and lower back, but can appear anywhere on your body. Most people are only affected with small patches. In some cases, the patches can be itchy or sore.

This disease lasts long term and can leave the sufferer with periods of no effect and times where it's severe. Anyone who suffers from this has to find their own individual way to calm down the symptoms, and studies have discovered that CBD slows down the production of keratinocytes in the epidermis of the skin, which is produced too quickly in people with psoriasis (*wayofleaf.com/cbd/ailments/cbd-for-psoriasis*).

It has also been found that CBD oil has significant soothing properties. Its substantial skin-calming and skin-normalizing effects can help minimize issues related to skin sensitivity, including redness and reactivity.

Dosage: This will depend on the severity of your condition. Consult a medical professional first as they will be able to give you the correct advice according to your individual needs.

Application: Oil, or topically applied to the affected area.

Precautions: Be aware of the side effects, which can include low blood pressure and dry mouth.

45. *Hair Issues*

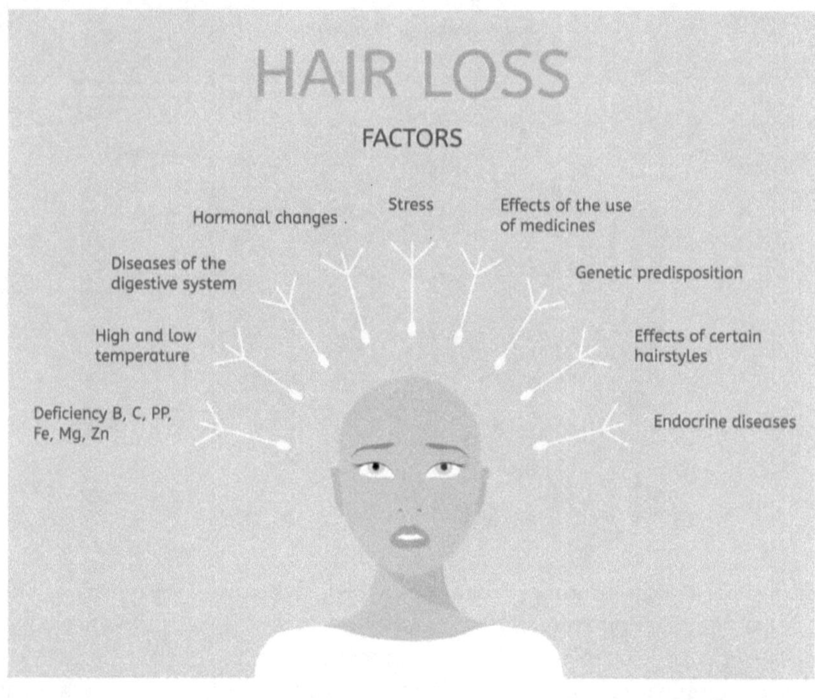

Hair loss is normal. We all lose an average of 50 to 100 hairs a day, usually without even thinking about it. However, if it's more than that, or if it's coming out in clumps leaving bald patches and burns behind, then **it could be because of:**

- Iron deficiency

- Medication or treatment

- Sickness

- Stress

- Weight loss

Studies have found that CBD oil increases blood circulation (*ncbi.nlm.nih.gov/pmc/articles/PMC3579247*), which has an effect on hair loss when used directly on the hair follicles because it helps to deliver nutrients stimulating hair growth. Many users have also found positive results on improving the condition of the hair. CBD oil not also reduces inflammation in the body, which can promote a healthier environment for hair to grow on the scalp, but is also suspected to reach sebaceous glands—which secrete oil (a.k.a. sebum) to lubricate hair—in hair follicles where it can provide therapeutic benefits.

TIP: If you see the cannabis plant on the label, that doesn't mean that the formula contains CBD oil. A lot of cannabis products on shelves usually contain hemp seed oil, which has the fatty acids that can help with moisturizing your hair, but do not have the same anti-inflammatory benefits that CBD oil for hair has. If you want to use CBD to optimize your chances for fuller, longer hair, consume full-spectrum CBD oil.

Dosage: There isn't a fixed dosage and it varies from individual.

Application: Oil, or topically applied to the hair. Start low and look for signs of improvement. You can also look at CBD-infused multivitamins for hair (e.g. *vegamour.com/products/gro-advanced-gummies-multi*).

Precautions: If it makes the symptoms worse, consult a medical professional.

46. *Bacteria*

Bacteria are microscopic, single-cell organisms that live almost everywhere. Bacteria live in every climate and location on earth. While many of these are harmless, there are some that can lead to sicknesses such as food poisoning, meningitis, and pneumonia to name a few.

Researchers have discovered that CBD has a built-in capacity to fight against such drug-resistant bacteria. One particular study (at *technologyreview.com/s/410815/a-new-mrsa-defense*) conducted by Giovanni Appendino (from Piemonte Orientale University, Italy) and Simon Gibbons (from the School of Pharmacy, University of London, U.K.) stated that: *"The cannabinoids even showed exceptional activity against the MRSA strain that makes extra amounts of the proteins that give the bugs resistance against many antibiotics. These proteins, he explains, allow the bacteria to 'hoover up unwanted things from inside the cell and spit them out again."*

Dosage: This will depend on the severity of your condition. Consult a medical professional first as they will be able to give you the correct advice according to your individual needs.

Application: Oil, capsules, or topically applied.

Precautions: Be aware of the side effects, which can include drowsiness, digestive issues, and low blood pressure.

47. Oxidative Stress

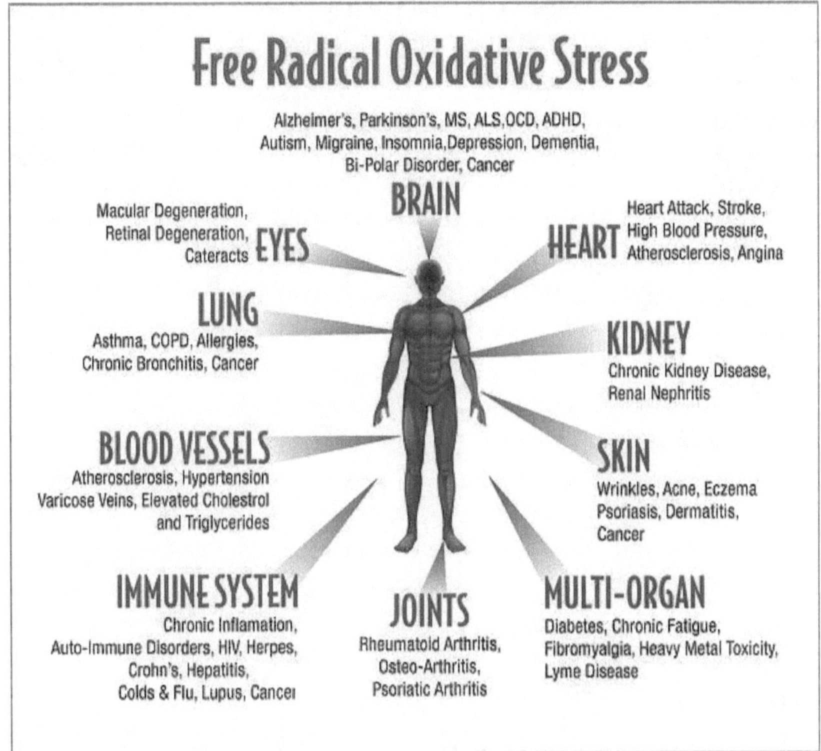

Oxidative stress is essentially an imbalance between the production of free radicals and the ability of the body to counteract or detoxify their harmful effects through neutralization by antioxidants. Stress on the body can lead to illnesses and diseases developing.

The potential symptoms are listed as:

- Brain fog and/or memory loss

- Decreased eye sight

- Fatigue

- Joint and/or muscle pain

- Sensitivity to noise and headaches

- Susceptibility to infections

- Wrinkles and grey hair

There have been many studies to suggest that the use of CBD oils can reverse the effects of this stress by replacing the body's antioxidants and the nutrients that might be missing in a person's diet (*pub-*

med.ncbi.nlm.nih.gov/20561509).

Dosage: Start with 25 mg of CDB oil per day. Some studies show that other hemp products may be also beneficial (_pubmed.ncbi.nlm.nih.gov/25493943_).

Application: Oils or capsules.

Precautions: Consult a medical professional first to find the underlying cause. Also be aware of the side effects, which can include drowsiness and dry mouth.

48. Weight Problems

Obesity is a medical condition in which excess body fat has accumulated to the extent that it may have a negative effect on health. You can discover what your ideal body weight is by using the Body Mass Index calculator available online, which employs your height and weight to see what percentage your body fat is of your body weight.

Did you know that according to National Health and Nutrition Examination Survey, 2 out of 3 people in America are either overweight or obese?

Obesity has many potential side effects, including pain, fatigue, certain types of cancer, heart disease, and diabetes, which, of course, are very serious. This is why you must make changes right away. You can treat it by eating a balanced diet, exercising, and living much healthier.

Studies have found that CBD may help reducing the appetite and the risk to insulin resistance levels, lower blood sugar levels, and high blood pressure, while also regulating the endocannabinoid system (*ncbi.nlm.nih.gov/pmc/articles/PMC6163475*). This assists users in losing weight and maintaining a healthy body mass index. Another study found that CBD has helped convert white fat cells into brown fat cells, which stimulates the body to break down fats more efficiently.

TIP: Always choose Full-Spectrum CBD Oil for weight loss rather than CBD isolates, because the other chemicals found in the plant makes it more effective.

Dosage: Start with 5-10 mg of CBD oil per day and increase for desired effects (*cbdoil.blog/cbd-weight-loss-faqs*).

Application: Oils, capsules, or gummies.

Precautions: Be aware of the side effects, which can include fatigue, stomach issues, and dry mouth.

49. *Glaucoma*

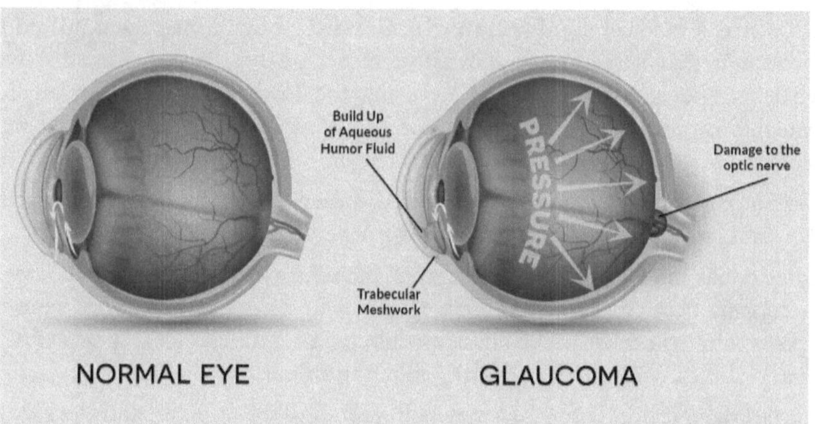

Glaucoma is an eye condition where your optic nerve is damaged by the pressure of the fluid inside your eye. Most types of glaucoma have no symptoms, so a regular eye test is the only way to know you have the condition. Treatment with drops can often prevent glaucoma causing sight loss. It can be caused by old age, other medical conditions, or family history.

Here is **the list of the symptoms**:

- Blurred vision

- Intense eye pain

- Headache

- Nausea and vomiting

- Red eyes

- Tenderness around the eyes

- Seeing rings around lights

If this is something you suspect you might have, you need to get medical help immediately because the longer you leave it, the worse it will become.

Studies have found that when using CBD as an eyedrop, the pressure on the eye is released which alleviates the symptoms and slows the progression (*leafly.com/news/health/cannabis-for-glaucoma-treatment*).

Dosage: A single sublingual CBD oil dose of 20-40 mg of CBD directly into eyes. Amounts larger than 40 mg per day could increase eye pressure.

Application: Topically to the eye.

Precautions: Consult a medical professional first with regards to your current healthcare plan. It can slow down the effects of your current medication. You may also experience drowsiness.

50. *Tinnitus*

Tinnitus is the name for hearing noises that aren't caused by an outside source. It's not usually a sign of any serious conditions and generally improves over time. These sounds can be ringing, buzzing, whooshing, humming, throbbing, or music. The sounds can be heard in one or both ears or in your head.

It is suggested that **the most common causes** for this are:

- Cardiovascular diseases

- Diabetes

- Ear infections

- Earwax or a foreign object touching the eardrum

- Middle ear (eustachian tube) issues

- Neck and head injuries

- Stiff middle ear bones

- TMJ (temporomandibular joint) disorders

- Traumatic brain injury

So, it is always advisable to seek out a medical opinion to confirm it isn't something more serious.

People who have used CBD for this have reported different results. Some have said that it gets rid of the side effects of the illness, e.g., anxiety, and others suggest it got rid of the noise completely and almost right away (*tinnitustalk.com*). So, it's worth a try to see if it affects you positively.

Dosage: Start with 25 mg of CBD oil per day and increase if needed.

Application: Oil.

Precautions: Be aware of the side effects, which can include drowsiness, dizziness, and diarrhea.

FAQS

1. *Is CBD oil a medicine?*

While CBD oil is not officially a medicine, there have been many studies into its usefulness. It's an alternative or complementary medicine, however; so when taking it, you should treat it as you would a traditional medication. Get advice from a medical professional to check if it suits you.

2. *Are there any side effects of CBD oil?*

There are potential side effects that you need to be aware of:

- Drowsiness
- Dry mouth
- Increase in tremors for some Parkinson's patients
- Inhibited hepatic drug metabolism and/or reduced effectiveness of p-glycoprotein and other drug transporters
- Light-headedness
- Low blood pressure

If you notice anything that doesn't quite feel right after taking CBD, then please consult your doctor.

3. *What is the difference between CBD oil and hemp oil?*

They are made from different parts of the plant. Hemp oil comes from pressing the plant's seeds, whereas CBD uses more of the plant. It can also be derived from hemp or cannabis plants.

4. *Can CBD oil help me with my pain?*

As written in this guide, CBD has been shown to have a massive positive effect in patients who suffer from pain (*medicalnewstoday.com/articles/319475*). Just be sure to confirm that it'll work well with your other medications too.

5. Is CBD oil safe to use?

There is no THC in a CBD product, making it safe to use, as long as you've consulted a doctor first. It's always better to buy from a reputable company to get the best, safest product for your money.

6. Can CBD oil help me with my anxiety?

A lot of work has been done with anxiety sufferers to confirm a very positive reaction. By working on the receptors in the nervous system, it calms users down (*leafly.com/news/health/how-to-use-cbd-for-anxiety*).

7. How long does CBD take to work?

There are a number of factors that determine how long it takes for the oil to take effect. Mostly the dosage and the ailment being treated. It's also individual to how receptive your body is.

8. Can CBD oil help me with my depression?

CBD oil might not be able to cure depression, but it can help to alleviate the symptoms by working with the endocannabinoid system. It helps to regulate essential human functions such as sleep, mood, pain, appetite, and pleasure.

9. Can CBD oil be toxic?

CBD oil is a nontoxic product, but there are studies being conducted all the time to ensure that the most up to date information is available.

10. Why is CBD oil so expensive?

The cost of CBD oil also needs to cover the cost of research. Because this isn't government funded, the companies have to keep on top of it.

11. Is CBD oil legal?

In most places, CBD oil is legal, but for information on where you live, check out the earlier chapter about the legal status of this oil in the world.

12. Is it legal to grow your own hemp?

It can be legal to grow your own hemp, depending on where you live. But you might need a license, so it's best to do some research into this first. To get you started, *The National Agricultural Law Center* (at *nationalaglawcenter.org*) has a guide to where it's legal to grow hemp right now.

13. Why are there legal restrictions on CBD?

Cannabidiol is not a controlled substance, but because of its link to cannabis, there can be some tricky issues. It's always best to buy from a reputable supplier and to speak to a medical professional to ensure that you have the most up to date information on your side.

14. *Does CBD make you high or show up on a drug test?*

No, without the THC, CBD will not get you 'high,' nor will it show up on drug tests. It contains none of the illegal substances, so you won't have any issues using it.

15. *Can CBD oil help diabetes in any way?*

One of the most common side effects of diabetes is chronic inflammation, which CBD can help with. It'll also be beneficial in assisting the immune systems, cell growth, sugar metabolism, and heart function – all of which is extremely useful for a sufferer of diabetes.

GLOSSARY OF TERMS

Here is **a glossary of terms** that is useful for talking about hemp and CBD:

Cannabinoids: Chemical compounds found in the cannabis plant but not in other plants. Of the dozens of cannabinoids identified so far, the most common are tetrahydrocannabinol (THC) and cannabidiol (CBD).

Cannabinol: A compound whose derivatives, which include tetrahydrocannabinol (THC), are the active ingredients of cannabis.

Cannabidiol (CBD): Some scientific research has suggested that CBD is an effective anti-inflammatory that might have potential as a treatment for certain neurological conditions, including seizures. Because this form of medical marijuana is weak and doesn't deliver the "high" that regular marijuana does, it was nicknamed "Hippie's Disappointment."

Charlotte's Web: This variety is sometimes called "Hippie's Disappointment" due to its failure to deliver the customary "high" associated with regular marijuana. But because of Charlotte's Web's ability to reduce or stop seizures, hundreds of families with epileptic children have, in recent years, moved to Colorado to try oil made from the Charlotte's Web. This variety is named after a 5-year-old girl, Charlotte, whose seizures virtually halted after she began taking the product.

Controlled Substances Act (federal): Title 21 of the U.S. Code. The Controlled Substances Act (CSA) establishes five "schedules" – I through V – of controlled substances; those listed under Schedule I are considered as having the most potential for abuse. "Marihuana," as the word is spelled in the CSA, is listed immediately after lysergic acid diethylamide (LSD).

DEA Schedule I drug: From the Controlled Substances Act, Schedule I: (A) a drug or other substance is considered as having a high potential for abuse, (B) a drug or other substance is considered as having no currently accepted medical use for treatment in the United States, (C) lacks accepted safety for a person's use of the drug or other substance under medical supervision.

Endocannabinoid: The biological system within humans (and other animals) that serves as a cannabinoid receptor and allows them to feel the effects of marijuana.

Flower: The crystal-covered buds that are harvested, then dried, to be used as medication.

HB 307: House Bill 307, signed on March 25, 2016, by Florida Governor Rick Scott. This bill expanded the state's medical-marijuana law. The standing law had already provided exemptions for a small group of patients, under certain conditions, from facing criminal charges for using marijuana that has low THC content (less than 0.8%) but high cannabidiol (CBD) content. This expanded law now grants patients access to other forms of medical marijuana – under the condition that the patient is expected to die within 1 year without the use of life-sustaining procedures. This new law, however, continues to impose excessive requirements on doctors and is not expected to help many people who are terminally ill.

Imported hemp: Products such as hemp granola and hemp shampoo violate, technically, federal drug laws. But such products are sold in some health-food stores because imported hemp has generally been permitted into the United States – as it contains less than 0.3% THC.

Industrial hemp: Cannabis, with less than 0.3% THC, whose fibers are very strong. Industrial hemp is grown for use in, say, paper, textiles, and military applications.

Kief: This is the cannabis resin trichomes that can accumulate in containers or that may be sifted from loose, dry flowers through a mesh screen or sieve.

Phytocannabinoids: Oxygen-containing compounds derived from cannabis plants. Extensive research has been conducted on two phytocannabinoids: CBD (cannabidiol) and THC (tetrahydrocannabinol). CBD is not intoxicating and contains neuroprotective, anti-psychotic, anti-inflammatory, and anti-convulsive properties. THC has anti-inflammatory, anti-spasmodic, anti-tremor, and appetite-boosting properties.

Psychoactive constituent: Any substance that alters the user's brain functions. THC is the principal psychoactive constituent in marijuana. The most widely consumed psychoactive substance is coffee.

Recreational marijuana: Commonly called "weed" or "pot," recreational marijuana has a THC (tetrahydrocannabinol) level of about 15%.

Rosin: A method that uses heat and a flat mechanism to "press" out terpene- and cannabinoid-rich resin from cured marijuana flowers.

"Seed to sale" tracking: Used by medical-marijuana dispensaries, growers, and government agencies, this system tags and numbers plants. As each part of the cannabis plant is used – including the leaves, the stem, and any waste – that part is given its own serial number. In states where medical marijuana is legal, some software systems send data automatically to the state government.

SFO (solventless flower oil) rosin: SFO is made directly from the flowers of the cannabis plant; the process preserves the flowers' natural terpenes. These are the compounds that give each strain of cannabis its unique smell and taste.

Spice: Also known as "K2," "spice" is a generic term for synthetic cannabis.

Supermajority: More than a simple majority. When Florida put a medical-marijuana initiative on the 2014 ballot, it narrowly lost with 57.6% (Florida law requires a 60% supermajority).

Synthetic cannabinoids: Man-made versions of cannabis that are, chemically, different from cannabis but that affect the same brain receptors as tetrahydrocannabinol (THC). They include dronabinol and nabilone. Both are applied to alleviate nausea and vomiting triggered by chemotherapy.

Terpenes: The natural oils secreted by trichomes (small glands on the flowers and main fan leaves of mature cannabis plants). Terpenes impart distinctive flavors (citrus, mint, etc.) to the cannabis.

THC: Tetrahydrocannabinol is the active ingredient in marijuana that, depending on its concentration, produces the mind-altering effects.

Therapeutic hemp: Cannabis strains such as Charlotte's Web that provide relief from, for example, seizures or nausea.

Tincture: A liquid extract that can be ingested orally.

Topical: A medicine that is applied directly to some part of the body.

Trichomes: Small glands on the flowers and main fan leaves of mature cannabis plants; trichomes consist mainly of a stalk and a head. Cannabinoids such as tetrahydrocannabinol (THC) are produced in the heads.

CONCLUSION

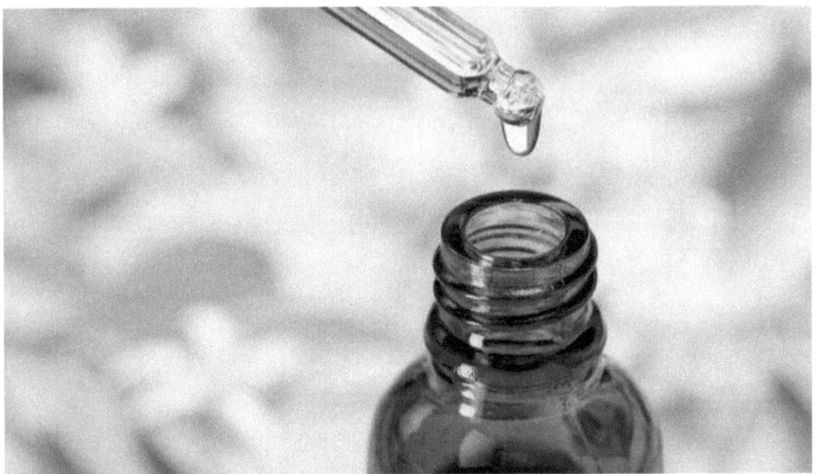

So, as you can see from this guide, there are a great number of ailments that CBD oil can help you with. There are only 50 listed; there are many more. If there's something you're curious about, then you can easily do your own research online. It's always advisable to do this anyway because the more you know about treating your own conditions, the better that treatment will be.

The **main benefits of CBD oil** can be found in:

- Pain management
- Anxiety and depression
- Heart, kidney, and liver health
- Neurological disorders
- The side effects of many illnesses

There are also many studies that keep giving you the most up to date research, so you will always be learning more.

Why not give CBD oil a try yourself to see what effect it can have on you and your condition? There are many places where you can get a sample, so there's no reason not to give it a go. Who knows, the positive side effects might make a real difference your life!

ABOUT THE AUTHOR

Mary Jones became interested in herbal remedies early on in her life. After becoming frustrated with the ineffectiveness and sometimes severe side effects of synthetic remedies, she started researching whether or not natural cures could be made to the same effect, without the use of synthetic means. After dedicating years of her life to research, learning from natural remedies masters, as well as from doctors that use natural cures to help their patients, she decided it was time to share the knowledge she had gathered with the world.

One of Mary's life goals is to make the world a better, happier place, and her writings are definitely a testament to that. She does not want to keep all of her research and discoveries to herself. She has elected to share them, in a format that makes them available to just about everyone. And instead of talking about just the unknown or difficult to find herbs, as many naturalists do, she has selected remedies that anyone can make, so that every person can make themselves healthier, easily and inexpensively. Mary's books aren't just about theory; they are about practice – actually fighting infections and ailments naturally!